Anders Bortne is an author and musician who has written five acclaimed books and released eight albums. He also works as a speechwriter for the Norwegian Minister of Justice. His debut novel was *A Good Band*, published in 2005. His third, *The Ice Man*, was nominated for The Youth Critic's Prize in 2011. Bortne's work observes both the extraordinary and the trivial, and frequently revolves around family and identity.

Lucy Moffatt is an award-winning translator from both Norwegian and Spanish into English. Born in London she now lives on the southern coast of Norway.

SLEEPLESS

ANDERS BORTNE

Translated
by
LUCY MOFFATT

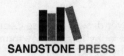

SANDSTONE PRESS

First published in Great Britain by
Sandstone Press Ltd
Willow House
Stoneyfield Business Park
Inverness
IV2 7PA
Scotland

www.sandstonepress.com

This translation has been published
with the financial support of NORLA.

ISBN: 978-1-913207-06-9
ISBNe: 978-1-913207-07-6

Sandstone Press is committed to a sustainable future. This book
is made from Forest Stewardship Council © certified paper.

Cover design by Rose Cooper
Typeset by Iolaire, Newtonmore
Printed and bound by CPI Group (UK) Ltd, Croydon, CR0 4YY

CONTENTS

'Without belabouring the point, insomnia is one of the most pressing and prevalent medical issues facing modern society, yet few speak of it this way, recognise the burden or feel there is a need to act.'

Matthew Walker
Sleep scientist and professor of neuroscience and psychology, in his book, *Why we Sleep*.

To all those who sleep.
And all those who do not.

INTRODUCTION

This book was written to help people with serious sleep problems, but it offers neither *a programme* nor concrete advice – like eating bananas or meditating before bedtime. This is the story of a sleepless life, but it is also an account of humanity's relationship with sleep. How did we sleep in earlier times? What happens when we sleep? And the most important question if you struggle with sleep yourself, or know somebody else who does: is there a solution that works?

After sixteen years my own sleep difficulties worsened, almost overnight and without my understanding why. A problem that I'd been able to live with was no longer manageable. I had to do something or go under. I embarked on the regular round of treatments that most insomniacs know only too well: pills, herbs, meditation, acupuncture, yoga. At the same time I started to read books about sleep and sleep difficulties – not just self-help books but clinical, psychological and historical texts about sleep. I couldn't find a single book aimed at people with serious sleep difficulties. Most of the books were written for people who were able to sleep but had opted out of it; or people who didn't understand that they ought to sleep more. Insomnia was, at best, a sub-chapter. And all the well-meaning but superficial sleep advice was, of course, no cure for a serious, chronic health problem. The most remarkable thing of all was the fact that we continue to veil sleep and sleep difficulties in mystery. Science – and people in general – have never known more about body and health; why do we treat sleep as if there were something mysterious about it?

I am not a doctor or a sleep expert. On the contrary: this book was written by a person who has suffered insomnia for many years and still sleeps poorly. If you are looking for a book that offers superficial tips about how to sleep better – drink less coffee, exercise more, set aside an hour during the day for your worries and so on – keep looking.

But perhaps you'd rather read this book, learn a bit about sleep and sleeplessness along the way, put two and two together for yourself and gain an insight into how other insomniacs are getting by.

If you ask me, you can't expect much more from a book.

Anders Bortne, Oslo,
30 January 2019

2

APRIL

Pills

About doctor's appointments and sleep medicine, facts and superstitions about sleep, how my problems started sixteen years ago and why insomniacs don't make pancakes.

I

Of course, the night before I'm due to see the doctor, I sleep like a log. I wake up rested. I'm not sweating and I'm not freezing. My head is clear. My muscles and joints aren't aching. Should I cancel? I don't like going to the doctor. I don't like sitting opposite a stranger revealing my own weaknesses. As long as I don't have anything solid to refer to – fever, or a wound or a broken bone – I'm afraid the whole thing will be reduced to feelings. *I can't sleep.* Now I've slept, though. I feel better than I have in a long time.

I meet my own gaze in the waiting room mirror: steady and clear. My skin has that faint glow I envy other people on sleepless days – a sign of health, of normality, of a night of long, deep sleep.

Maybe I'm cured?

Maybe it's over at last?

That wasn't what I thought a week ago, when I made the doctor's appointment. I was standing over the bed I share with Line changing the bedclothes – a job nobody

3

but me is allowed to do. Just as a person with eating disorders can become obsessed with the fridge, I'm fixated on the conditions surrounding my own bed. Pillowcases and duvet covers must have buttons to prevent their innards oozing out in the middle of the night. The mattress protector cannot have a single crease or unevenness. If any clothes or other items are lying on the bed when I'm about to go to sleep, I have to go out again and make another attempt later. The cables of the bedside lamps must be firmly secured to the wall to stop them knocking against the panel when somebody moves. The mere *thought* that the light bulb in the lamp might be too bright can ruin the night for me.

As I tugged off the sheet, the sun shone through the basement window, through the swirling dust and down onto the mattress protector. I stopped and stood there staring at the naked bed as the hairs rose on the back of my neck. I had changed the bedclothes many times, but I'd never noticed this before: on the left-hand side, Line's side, I could see wear and tear in the fabric that bore witness to a life of normal night-time sleep. It was many years since we'd bought the bed; of course, it would be worn. But on the other side of the bed, my side, there wasn't a mark. The mattress protector looked untouched. It was as if my wife had shared her bed with a ghost all these years.

For all my obsession with the bed, I hardly lay in it at all.

I dropped the bedclothes, sat down on the mattress and did something I'd never done before. I pulled out my mobile and googled *sleep deprivation* and *long-term effects*, then clicked my way to an internet article entitled: 'Here is the terrifying list of what sleep deprivation can lead to'. Diabetes, it said. High cholesterol levels.

Stroke, heart attack. Cancer. Beneath the list was a fact box detailing how many hours you needed to sleep each night to maintain your health. It said adults need seven to eight hours' sleep every night.

I got scared and made a doctor's appointment.

The next day, I was no longer frightened and wanted to cancel. I knew that the fear would return. My own feelings tracked my sleep problems and the sleep problems came and went. I fell sick, I was cured; I fell sick again and was cured again. Right now I was no longer sick, I had slept well the night before – so I wasn't afraid. There was nothing a general practitioner could help me with anyway, so why waste my time?

'That doctor's appointment,' I said to Line. 'I think I'll cancel.'

She looked at me.

'Are you sure?'

'The only thing a doctor can do is give me sleeping pills. And I don't want those.'

'But if you want any other help, you'll have to start with the doctor anyway.'

In the waiting room at the doctor's surgery a woman with crutches and a neck brace sits opposite me, gaze fixed helplessly on the ceiling. Beside me waits an older man who emits a deep rattling cough every twenty seconds. Over by the door, a mother tries to get a newborn child to stop crying. In the midst of all this, I sit there, well rested and healthy, hoping I won't get called in before the others.

Then the doctor comes out.

'Bortne?'

My little speech comes out more or less as planned. 'I've had chronic insomnia for sixteen years,' I start. The

5

medical book I borrowed from the library a couple of days ago used the official Norwegian term *insomni* not the widely used English variant, *insomnia*, but since I'm afraid he'll think I've read myself ill – and besides I want him to be the person in the room who knows most about the subject – I use the more popular, albeit less correct variant.

'Lately my insomnia has got worse. And now I'm starting to worry about the long-term effects of getting too little sleep. I'm also worried about my heart. And about getting cancer.'

I detail the fear I felt a week ago, try to hold it firm for long enough to describe it to the other person even though it feels as if I'm lying.

'I have to find out why I don't sleep,' I say. 'Maybe there isn't a single explanation, maybe there are many causes. I'm willing to give most things a try. I'm no longer looking for a quick fix.'

I meet the doctor's gaze. A young man – younger than me anyway – with dark curls and round, black-framed spectacles. He is the locum of the locum of my GP, whom I've never met. His face is blank, expressionless. Maybe he's used to patients seeing him as an obstacle between them and their medicine. But I don't want to be sent home with sleeping pills. I'd rather go home and carry on as before.

The doctor spreads his fingers over his keyboard and writes down some of what I say before placing his hands in his lap and listening again.

'I try to deal with it by myself, too,' I say.

'How do you do that?'

My phone rings. I quickly fish it out of my inside pocket and reject the call.

'I've stopped surfing the net, I've signed out of

Facebook, I try to read more books, force my brain to think long thoughts. I've bought myself a diary. I've started exercising. And I try to put down my mobile telephone.'

My phone rings again.

'And how's that working for you?' asks the doctor.

I take it out and switch it off as I mumble an apology.

'I'm trying to learn a bit about sleep and sleep disorders,' I say. 'I've borrowed a medical book from the library.'

The doctor's gaze is on his screen; he doesn't look at me. I regret telling him that last bit. It was true: I'd gone to the library at lunchtime and borrowed a book called *Sleep and Sleep Disorders*, and I've read about the stages of sleep and circadian rhythm, about insomnia and other sleep problems. But why do I feel the need to tell the doctor about it?

I need to be careful, I think. Let doctors be doctors and patients be patients.

'Do you have difficulty getting to sleep?' he asks – it sounds as if he's reading from the screen. 'Or is it that you wake up too early and can't get back to sleep, or do you wake up a lot in the middle of the night?'

I give this some thought. It is difficult to see it like this, from the outside, with the doctor. In the early years, sleeplessness was just that: an ailment, a sickness, something observable. But in the past six or seven years, it has been *me*. I think back over the recent weeks. Last night I slept well, but the night before? I didn't sleep then. Or the night before, or the two nights before that. It is so difficult to remember: the sleepless nights and days merge, nothing stands out, there is nothing to navigate by. Like a long, dark tunnel: you only know when it begins and when it ends. Was it worse than before?

Was that why I'd got so scared? Was that why Line had insisted I should go?

'All three?' asks the doctor.

I nod.

'Have you noticed any other issues apart from sleep?'

'It's been very up and down for a while,' I say. 'But I'm used to it. I get a bit angry. Or wound up. Or down.'

I tried to avoid the word *mood*.

'Do you work?'

'Yes.'

'What do you do?'

'I work in a ministry, as a speechwriter. And I'm an author too. I also have a cartoon strip in a newspaper. And I'm involved in a couple of music projects as well.'

'Sounds like a lot,' says the doctor.

'A few weeks ago, I had to take time off sick. I couldn't take any more. It's the first time I've been off sick because of sleep.'

'How long were you off?'

'Four days.'

A bug, is what I told my boss. If I'd told them the truth, that I was off sick because I could no longer cope with my own insomnia, they'd have started wondering what was *really* wrong with me. I don't hide my sleep problems, but so far, it's something I haven't tended to share with people who aren't close to me. Saying *I don't sleep* is like saying *I'm bleeding* – everybody will wonder what caused it. And since I don't have a good answer, anybody can fill in the blanks for themselves. Anders is depressed, Anders has experienced some trauma, Anders is unhappy in his job or his home life or both. Until I've found the answer for myself, I'm afraid other people will see me as weak.

I don't know why I bleed: I just do.

Taking sick leave, even for a few days, was a defeat. When it appeared sixteen years ago, my insomnia was like a huge rock that had dropped into the middle of the road, but I always managed to find a way around it: I'd go home at lunchtime to sleep, come in an hour later, leave an hour earlier, or simply hold out until I could sleep again. This wasn't the first time I'd been stopped in my tracks by my sleep difficulties; but I'd never taken sick leave before because of sleep deprivation. I couldn't fight my way forward any more. There was no way around.

'Have you tried a sleep study?' asks the doctor.

'No,' I say. 'Do you think it would be any use?'

Sleep study is a term that has popped up in the past few years on the few occasions when I've talked about my sleep problems with friends or family. *Have you tried a sleep study?* Was this my great hope? Was that why I was here? I wasn't even sure what it was, other than it involved spending a night sleeping at a hospital and being watched. It sounded like an insomniac's PhD thesis: *Sleep study*.

The doctor shoves himself away from his desk, so that his chair trundles across the floor towards a shelf where he pulls down a thin folder, which looks like his own notes. He searches in the folder, reads a bit, continues searching. The last time I was here with one of my kids, he didn't meet my gaze once. I'm used to doctors who've seen everything, heard everything, who never quite believe that there's anything seriously wrong, regardless of what ailment you come in with. But now he's curious and engaged. Maybe I'm the day's most interesting patient. Maybe he's only had migraine and flu cases today, and in I sail with sixteen years' worth of insomnia. Maybe cases like mine were what made him take up medicine in the first place. Maybe he'll start to flip through folders from his student days, ring his old professor, who also awakens from his academic slumber to ring him back in the middle of the night with suggestions for ground-breaking solutions. Overtime food, blackboards full of scientific formulae, late nights in the library basement.

'I don't know,' he says, still bent over his folder. 'But it's normal to look for underlying causes.'

'What do you mean?'

'Well, what's stopping you sleeping. There can be a lot of reasons, as you said yourself. Perhaps a sleep study will help identify them.'

He shuts the folder, puts it back where he found it and shoves himself back to his PC.

As a result of telling my doctor about my problems, of asking him for help, I now feel something I haven't felt for a long time: hope. Hope and fear. Do the two always go together? Is that why I was so reluctant to go to the doctor? Was I afraid to start hoping again?

'But in the meantime, I have something I think might work,' he says. 'They're not sleeping pills but a medication that's used for bipolar disorders.'

'Do you think I'm bipolar? Is that why I'm not sleeping?'

'It doesn't sound as if you have a bipolar disorder. You function at work and a few flare-ups now and then don't qualify. But it isn't unusual to use medicines that are intended for one purpose for something quite different. And this one can be used to sleep. What it does is suppress your thought processes.'

'It stops the thought processes?'

'It suppresses them, for the night.'

'So it's not like I'll turn into a vegetable?'

'No, these are sleeping pills.'

I nod but I don't understand. Are they sleeping pills or not? What I fear most of all is taking medication that reduces or eliminates my capacity to write or make music. If I lose that, it's irrelevant whether I'm functioning in all other respects.

'How long should I take it for?'

'A week. Come back to see me after that. Then we can talk about how it's gone and I can look into the possibility of sending you for a sleep study.'

He writes out a prescription and indicates that the appointment is over. 'Don't be alarmed by what it says on the packaging,' he says as I leave his office.

When I'm in the chemists a few hours later picking up the medicine, I discover that my bankcard isn't in my wallet. I must have left it at work. I cycle to the office, find the card on my desk, cycle back to the chemists and breathlessly wave the card at the woman behind the counter, who smiles aloofly. I, who had decided not to resort to medicine, who went to the doctor in search of a lasting solution – here I stand in front of the pharmacist like an idiot, rejoicing:

Look, I can pay for my pills!

The pharmacist pushes the box of pills across the counter and keys the amount into the till. I swipe my card. The box looks like any other medicine: a flat, white, rectangular cardboard box.

'Don't be alarmed by what it says on the packaging,' she says.

I pick up the kids from nursery, put them in the bike trailer and cycle home. As they play outside, I cook tomato soup, fry some pancakes and invite the little girl next door to have dinner with us. After eating, I run upstairs to the family above us with the remaining pancakes. If I'd slept badly last night, we would have been sitting here with ham pizza and cola. The neighbours would have had to fend for themselves. But now I have the energy to behave like a properly functioning, resourceful human being.

Line is working late and won't get home until the kids are in bed. I tell her about the doctor's appointment and the medicine I've been given.

'But that was what you didn't want,' she says. 'You said so yourself, that you'd decided you didn't want to have sleeping pills.'

'But these aren't sleeping pills,' I say.

'Aren't they?'

'The doctor says they suppress your thought processes. He wants to see if they work on me.'

Line looks at me. I can see she has her own opinion but doesn't want to say any more. It's my decision. I put the box of pills on the table between us, unfold the thin paper containing information about the medicine until it is the size of an average tablecloth and read.

Antipsychotic. For schizophrenia and mania and bipolar disorders.

II

The sleeplessness arrived in my late twenties, coinciding with the end of my studies, my move from Bergen to Oslo and starting work. Every morning I went to work and in the afternoons I practised with my two bands. In the evenings I went out with friends. At the weekends I worked on my first novel. My social network was large and my ambitions were sky-high. And in the midst of all this, I met Line.

I lived in a filthy little two-room apartment right at the bottom of Trondheimsveien – the first place I'd had all to myself. I remember loving that flat, even though I now remember it as the place where my sleeplessness began. In the little bedroom, on an Ikea box mattress, I started lying awake all through the night: I'd hear the last tram racketing past at one in the morning and the early morning tram at five o'clock. In the mornings, I'd sit shivering on the edge of my bed filled with an unease I didn't understand. Nothing had happened, nothing would happen. I would be doing the same things I'd done the day before: shower, get dressed, brush my teeth and go to work, where I would write articles for the postal service's internal bulletin. The most dramatic part of my job was taking pictures of the employee of the month receiving a giant cardboard cheque. What was I so afraid of? Why wasn't I sleeping? I looked at myself in the mirror. It didn't show that I'd lain awake all night, and the days without sleep went surprisingly well. And I would sleep again that night, for sure.

But the sleep never came; it just carried on – two nights, three, four in a row.

I was so surprised by this sudden absence of sleep that I'd tell acquaintances I met about it, as if I'd been mugged in the middle of the street. *I haven't slept for two nights! It's true! I don't know what's causing it!*

I wasn't looking to understand *why* I wasn't sleeping; I simply needed to sleep. I went to the doctor – a different one in those days – who also prescribed sleeping pills. What else was there? Sleeping pills were the only things the doctor and I both knew about; of course I would take pills. And at first they worked. Imovane, Apodorm, Stilnoct. I went to the doctor and got the prescription, and when I ran out, I got a friend who was newly qualified and had his medical licence to write out prescriptions on evenings and weekends. Sometimes I got sleep medicine from friends who had some lying around at home. If my pill-pusher didn't have time to meet me, we'd agree a place where I could go and pick it up. I had the inventiveness and persuasive capacity of all pill addicts. I always managed to get hold of pills but simultaneously tried to hide how desperate I was. Once I arranged a meeting with a friend who said she had one pill at home. I hadn't slept for three nights and had no other options. She was due to leave town, so I persuaded her to leave the pill in a plastic bag underneath the rubbish bins outside her apartment building before she left. Through the city in the pouring rain I walked to the agreed spot, lay down on the ground and fumbled beneath the rubbish bins until I found the plastic bag. Happily, I headed home, one hand in my pocket, clutching the crumpled pill package with its single remaining pill.

One little tablet and I slept at night. If I had to do something the next day that required me to be at my best, I could count on one of the little pills. By the time I published my first book, I was totally reliant on sleeping pills the night before an interview. I was terrified of sitting there like a zombie: I wanted to give the impression of being smart, clever, *alert*. And I came out better in the photos too.

This was before I realised my sleep problems were there to stay. For me, sleeplessness was a burden I would have to carry for a while, but which I would one day be able to set down. In the meantime, I did my best to hide its weight from other people, and to hold out. So, I took a pill, slept deeply, slept long and woke up fully rested the next day.

It was too good to last. The pills became less and less

effective and in the end they had zero effect. Instead I became woozy, apathetic, dry-mouthed.

Sleep medicine does not result in natural sleep. Studies have shown that people who sleep with the aid of sleeping pills don't get enough of the deepest brainwaves, which determine how deeply and well we sleep.[1] Sleeping pills attack the receptors, preventing brain cells from sending out impulses. They are sedatives – the pills anaesthetise you, just like alcohol – and are a bad foundation on which to build a lifestyle. And then there are the unintended effects of sleeping pills that I wasn't aware of when I was addicted myself – because I *was* addicted. Sleeping pills can make you forgetful; you can act without being fully conscious; your reaction time can increase the day after taking them, making you a dangerous driver. When you stop taking sleeping pills, you may end up sleeping more poorly than you did before you started taking them. And it gets worse. A large American study compared 10,000 patients who took sleeping pills with 20,000 people who didn't take medicine to help them sleep.[2] Those who took sleeping pills were 4.6 times more likely to die in the course of the two-and-a-half year study period. Mortality increased the more often people took the pills. The study also proved what earlier studies had suggested: that there was a link between sleeping pills and cancer. People who took sleep medicine had a 30–40 per cent higher likelihood of developing cancer!

Sleeping pills work badly and can kill you. But even though I know that now, I would still take sleeping pills regardless if I knew they helped. Wouldn't a person who hadn't had food for three days eat anything to allay their hunger, oblivious to warnings about potential side effects? When you can't sleep, you'll do anything for a few hours of sleep – just ask the half a million Norwegians who currently take sleeping pills. And the numbers are increasing. Between 2000 and 2012, usage of sleep medicine rose from 6.9 per cent to 11.1 per cent.[3]

I know only one other person who suffers what I suffer from, chronic insomnia. But almost everybody I know has tried sleeping pills at one time or another. And you don't need to search under rubbish bins for them the way I did. One friend started taking sleeping pills when he was hospitalised and has continued ever since. Every time he runs out, he logs on to his doctor's website and writes just two words: sleeping pills, and then the prescription arrives. No questions asked.

Although the effects abated, I continued to take pills for a couple of years, out of sheer desperation. I tried to cut out the sleep medicine for a while to flush out my system – only to prepare my body for a new round of pills. But it didn't help. I tried what are known as sleep-inducing drugs, which had even less of an impact but equally troublesome side effects. The medicine had turned against me. It was my brain telling me to stop. Three years after insomnia entered my life, I had to give up the pills. I was better off without, even though I slept even more poorly in the vacuum that followed – which rapidly prompted me to look for other things that might help me sleep. But sleeping pills I never touched again.

Today, it is over twelve years since I last tried using medicine to sleep. Should I start up again?

III

The night is approaching. I ring a friend who is a doctor and whose partner also has sleep difficulties. He has helped me before, with advice, with prescriptions. I give him a quick rundown of my encounter with the doctor and read out the patient information leaflet.

'What are you scared of?' he asks.

'This medicine is for mental illness. All I want to do is sleep. I don't want to take anything that will change me in some way.'

'He's given you a very low dose. It's worth a try. You have nothing to lose.'

At half past ten I swallow one of the little pills; usually this would be far too early for me: there would be no question of my getting to sleep now unaided. Still, I think, if I'm going to cheat anyway, I might just as well get a long night out of it. For once, I go to bed at the same time as Line, who quickly shuts her eyes and falls silent. One of the first things I learned about her was how good her relationship with sleep is – and how much sleep she needs. Even in the periods when I'm sleeping normally, she still seems to need twice as much sleep as me. Now I watch her doze off, now comes that little start, as though she were stumbling over a threshold. She lies in her usual position: on her side, arms crossed, duvet covering the lower half of her face with only her nose poking out. Not a sound. She sleeps, and she will sleep for many hours. She is borne away on the journey that all sleepers make every single night, consisting of the different stages of sleep: first dropping off, drowsing between the waking and sleeping state, then onward into the light sleep in which she will spend half the night. This is the level of sleep we return to whenever we have spent time in one stage and are about to make the transition to another. The brain no longer receives any sensory impressions. We sleep. After the first half hour, we descend into deep sleep, delta sleep. In deep sleep, the sensory doors are firmly shut. If the kids whimper or cry out, Line won't jump up, whereas I will, since I almost always seem to be in a lighter sleep. In deep sleep, there are no eye movements, the muscles are more relaxed, the brain's rhythm alters, and it starts to work in slow, deep waves, delta waves, at 0.5 to three cycles per second. It's like the activity in a swimming pool: when the pool is full of extremely active people, they create many small waves. If there are only a few people who are moving less but in time with one another, the waves are fewer but higher.[4] This is how the brain works when our surroundings are shut out for the night. After sleeping deeply for roughly one-and-a-half hours, we are brought back to the light sleep, but only for a few minutes, before entering REM sleep, which is distinct from the other stages. Here, the brainwaves become small and short again, our eyes move rapidly from side to side, our breathing becomes irregular and our muscles are paralysed. After spending a brief period in the night's first stage of REM sleep, the cycle is repeated: light sleep, deep sleep, light sleep, REM sleep; light sleep, deep sleep, light sleep, REM sleep. If we wake up during the night, it will probably be between these cycles, which are repeated until we awaken. But they will not be identical. As the night's sleep approaches its end, each cycle will contain less deep sleep and more REM sleep. Nearly all the deep sleep we get is in the first half of the night. Just before we wake, the REM stages will be at their longest.

Line sleeps. I, meanwhile, lie gazing out into the dark room, still wide awake, as I wait for an outside force, developed by a pharmaceutical firm and produced in a factory, to come and pull me into sleep. But for the knowledge that a little blue pill is dissolving inside me and dispatching its active ingredients into my blood and up to my brain, I would have got up again long ago. I don't want to let anything get in the way of the medicine, so I don't read, I don't play music or watch a film on my iPad. Instead, I do something I stopped doing many years ago: I just lie there, waiting.

Soon I notice a heaviness, as if I were being pressed down into the mattress and pillow; my arms and legs become leaden, my eyelids slide shut and I am dragged into something that resembles sleep.

Sleep isn't just a fundamental human state – it is where everything begins and ends. In sleep, the heart takes its first beat; in sleep, most hearts take their last beat. Sleep cocoons our lives, providing the merciful lulls in our existence. Our waking life stands on the shoulders of our sleeping hours. And yet the body and mind seem to do their utmost to keep the two separate. The person who is about to sleep shuts the door, draws the curtains and switches off the light, curling up beneath a blanket. Their face is hidden and their eyes are closed, as if nothing must be revealed to the waking world.

When did sleep evolve? We now know that all animals sleep – even insects – but has it always been this way? Worms emerged during the Cambrian explosion more than 500 million years ago; apparently, they took a nap from time to time.[5] We do not know how the dinosaurs slept, although people have found fossils of what appear to be sleeping dinosaurs. Mei long – Chinese for 'sleeping dragon' – is one of the most famous fossils, a troontid from the Cretaceous period, which was found in a posture akin to that of modern-day birds at rest: head hidden beneath its wing, hind legs tucked under its body.

Fourteen million years ago, all mammals still slept for short periods – often just minutes at a time. The Pierola apes, possibly early forebears of both humans and the large human apes, lived on the Iberian Peninsula and were the first primates to build nests in the treetops, which enabled them to sleep through the night without having to defend themselves against threats on the ground. This was the start of long, continuous night-time sleep[6]. Later, the species that would evolve into humans mastered fire, which enabled them to sleep long and safe on the ground. Our forebears' quest for a safe night's sleep prompted a new evolutionary direction. Longer periods of sleep also allowed us to achieve higher-quality sleep. The largest share, REM sleep or dream sleep in particular, has contributed to what we now acknowledge to be human qualities: plentiful, complex emotions and empathy, but also highly developed cognitive abilities, good memory and creativity. One might claim that prolonged sleep, above all, is what has made us human.

And yet, the divide between our sleeping and waking hours seems so unbridgeable. Sleep, like death, ensures that we cannot take anything into it with us. Or back from it. If we have had a meal, we can remember everything: how we sat at the table, how the food and drink were put in front of us, the appearance of the different dishes, aromas and tastes, what we ate, how much we put on our plates, what we liked and didn't like. Sleep, in contrast, is forgotten the moment we wake. We can remember being tired and going to bed. We no longer feel tired. We see that time has passed. But we have no memories of sleeping. Where have we been? What have we done? Sleep leaves no marks upon our bodies. No other traces, for that matter. Just look at human history:

everything we know today is based on humanity's waking state. About sleep and the night, we know next to nothing.

We can remember dreams, but if we don't process them in our consciousness, the impressions are erased in a matter of minutes. Sleep's endeavours to cover its tracks even encroach on our waking state. The last minutes *before* we doze off are wiped from our memory as we sleep. In other words, sleep's amnesia has a retroactive effect, as demonstrated by research [7]: test subjects were played short combinations of words as they fell asleep. Those who were woken thirty seconds after dozing off could still remember what was said up until the point when they fell asleep. But those who were woken after sleeping for ten minutes could not remember the words spoken in the final minutes before they fell asleep; some lacked memories from as far back as ten minutes before sleep came. The fact that we do not remember falling asleep, or the time before it, may also explain why we don't remember short periods of wakefulness during the night.

The impenetrable nature of sleep also seems to have cocooned human imagination on the topic. Mythology has always reflected humanity's principal fascinations. Pantheons have flourished in the realms of sex, war, death and intoxication. But when it comes to sleep, the myths are few and far between. In Norse mythology, there is no dedicated god of sleep; the nearest we get to it is Natt, the female Jotun – a type of giantess known as a *gyger*. Every night, she rides across the sky on her horse, Rimfakse, who leaves a trail of saliva behind him in the form of morning dew. In Greek mythology there is at least a separate god of sleep, Hypnos [8]. He is the twin brother of Thanatos, the god of peaceful death, a fact that tells us something about how the Greeks classified sleep. The god of sleep lives in his cave in Erebus, which, in Greek mythology, is a land of eternal darkness beyond the gates of the rising sun. Poppies grow outside Hypnos's cave and he wears a wreath of them around his head. Because Hypnos hates to be woken by noise, the cave has no creaking gates or doors. One of the five rivers of the underworld, the river of forgetfulness, flows past the sleep god's cave. From there, Hypnos cannot see whether it is day or night but that doesn't stop him from climbing up to the heavens every night with his mother Nyx, the goddess of night. In later European legends, sleep takes the form of a little man carrying a sack of magic sand that he sprinkles into people's eyes to make them sleep and dream. In Scandinavia, he is called Jon Blund or Ole Lukkøye, in Germany he is Sandmann and in English he is the Sandman. But he represents dreams, not sleep. It is easy to see why human imagination prefers dreams. Sleep itself is eventless. It is the hiatus, the blank intermission. In sleep, we are all abandoned to ourselves. Only in our dreams do we act and feel and through these actions and feelings we enter the interpersonal. Only in dreams can we see one another.

But to dream, you must sleep.

IV

Next morning, I sit up in bed. I feel dull and groggy. Did I sleep deeply enough? Long enough? Did I sleep at all? Over the years, I've become expert at observing and diagnosing my own sleep. And as with all other areas of expertise, the deeper you dig, the longer and more incomprehensible the answers become. It is a long time since I've given an honest answer to the question *Did you sleep well last night?* I have learned to simply nod and say *Pretty good.* The question is a pleasantry; nobody is asking for a dissertation.

Every day, I know roughly what awaits me, but I have no control over my nights. I never know what will happen and, as a rule, I don't know what has happened either. Sleep comes, or it does not. I may sleep the whole night through, or I may lie staring at the wall for an entire night. I may lie awake for half the night and sleep deeply for the other half. I may go to bed at three o'clock and start my day at 4.30am. I may spend eight hours in a kind of inert slumber without getting any deep sleep. I may have moved around, from bed to sofa number one, to sofa number two, to the floor in front of the TV and back to bed again. I may have watched three films. Some nights I find it, others not. Wherever sleep is, I try to follow.

At night, anything at all can happen, so the only thing I can do is sound myself out and try to put it into words.

But now I'm not sure.

I hear Line and the kids, who are awake and talking together up on the first floor. It's unusual for me to be the last person to wake up. I shower and dress, and as I cross the threshold from night to day I sense that something isn't right. Am I still feeling the effects of the pills? I must have been unconscious in some way or another but this doesn't feel like the aftertaste of sleep. I don't feel sleep-deprived, but I don't have that feeling of being recharged either, the way I do after a good night. When I come up to the first floor, my kids call out to me happily, but I can't summon up a smile.

'Morning,' Line says.

23

'Morning,' I reply.

The first words of the day, my first exchange with another human being – at times it's like opening the door to an overfilled cupboard. Some mornings, the contents stay in place; other times, everything comes tumbling out. This morning, I can tell I need to hold back: I have nothing worthwhile to offer. Hang in there, I think. In three-quarters of an hour, the kids will have been dropped off at kindergarten and I'll be at work. Work gives me the distance I need: distance from other people but also from myself. Here at home, with two small children, my life stares me in the face; there's no distance, no place to hide.

We start getting ready to leave the house. There are clothes and shoes to be found, drinking bottles and rain-coats to be remembered, bodies to be clothed. This is a situation in which I can quickly become impatient – this morning it is worse than ever. I start to sweat and then comes the itching. My chest contracts and I can't breathe. The hallway, with all these bodies and clothes and shoes, becomes like a cage for me. I just want to get out.

'But I don't want to wear jeans,' whines the five-year-old as I pull on her trousers. I feel the anger rising fast.

'You have to.'

'I don't *want* to.'

I hold her firmly. 'I couldn't care *less!*'

'Anders,' Line says reprovingly.

When we get out onto the doorstep, I grab hold of my two-year-old lad, who doesn't want to cross the threshold.

'Come here!'

He shakes his head.

'*Damn* it!' I bark, pulling him out into the sunlight. 'Come here!'

He gazes at me in astonishment.

'Daddy,' he says simply.

'You need to pull yourself together!' Line looks at me sternly and holds me with her gaze.

I'm hot and my back is damp, my scalp itchy. If I get angry, it's too late – I know that – but I don't *feel like* pulling myself together, I don't *feel like* holding back. Do the kids want to resist me every inch of the way? Does Line want an argument? Bring it on – I'm ready.

Now Line stops dead. It's as though she finds herself face to face with a stranger.

'What is the matter with you?' she says. 'Have you taken Dr Evil pills or something?'

I look at my kids' faces. The five-year-old is looking at me as if I were insane, while the two-year-old's face is red and contorted with weeping. I pick him up and try to comfort him, but he stretches his arms out to his mother, wriggling out of my embrace.

As I sit alone in the car after dropping the others off, I start to cry. It's as if the tears run down a mask: I can't feel them; I feel numb, leaden and medicated. My mouth is dry and there's a metallic taste on my tongue that I can't get rid of.

It's irrelevant whether these pills are meant to cure sleeplessness or misery. They don't work.

A week later, I'm standing in front of the mirror in the toilet at the doctor's surgery again. I lean over the sink and in towards the mirror. My eyes are glassy as if I were high or feverish. I go hot and cold in turn; my muscles and joints ache. Every time the kid at the play table in the corner slams his toy truck against the edge of the table, I jump. These symptoms aren't caused by the sleep medicine: they are my body's natural response to sleep deprivation. The previous night, I fell asleep early but woke up at one o'clock and couldn't get back to sleep. I didn't fall asleep until dawn, on the sofa. The night before it was just as bad.

Whether or not that one night of sleep medicine is what triggered a new bad patch I do not know. It's irrelevant. This has been going on for sixteen years. Sixteen years equals 5,840 nights. Assuming I ought to have slept seven hours per night that adds up to 40,880 hours I should have spent sleeping.

So many wakeful hours. So many lost hours.

I go back out into the waiting room, sit down, pick up an out-of-date women's magazine and find that the glossy paper is quivering between my fingers. An almost imperceptible tremor. I haven't noticed this before. Has the decline begun? Is age to blame, or is it all these years of sleep deprivation? What did it say in that article – was it a 40 per cent higher risk of getting cancer? More? Some nights, it felt as if my heart was galloping in my chest – what could that be? God almighty, how could I let this go on for so many years, just accepting all this sleep deprivation without doing anything about it? I have to try and find a solution. This isn't just about my health or my life; I have a family that needs me, healthy and strong and rested, for many years to come. Is it fear or hope that has brought me here again? Do the two always keep company?

My name is called and I shuffle into the doctor's office.

'How's it been going?' the doctor asks.

'No more pills,' I say. 'What else can I do to get some sleep?'

MAY

How To Sleep Better

About herbs, self-help books, meditation, psychiatry, hypnosis, coffee, yoga, masturbation and other good advice; what dreams actually are, a four-billion-year-old rhythm and how desperation will make you try everything twice.

I

You should try everything once. At lunch I go to the chemists – a different one this time: I don't want to be recognised, don't want to seem more desperate than I am, which just makes me seem even more desperate. Why am I trying to hide it? It's not as if I'm planning to poison anybody; I just want to sleep. I look for the section for over-the-counter remedies for sleep problems. Where does sleep belong? Is it classified under pain? Nutrition? In the end I approach the pharmacy technician. She shows me the shelf, which is under dietary supplements and contains a handful of products: Lifeline Care sleep capsules, which 'can help you relax, fall asleep more quickly and have better-quality sleep'; Valerina tablets 'for the relief of mild anxiety and sleep disorders'; and Pascoflair, whose blurb is concealed by a green label: 'New!' On the far left is a purple and white box labelled Sedix, 'for the relief of mild symptoms of anxiety and to aid sleep. Adults and children over 12.

Plant-based remedy'. In front of this last row of pillboxes is a blue sign: 'As Seen on TV'. It has been advertised on TV, the pharmacy technician explains. 'You know, they can advertise over-the-counter medication but not prescription drugs like sleeping pills. That's the doctors' domain. Every time a product is on TV, loads of people come in asking for it.'

'Do many people buy products like this? I mean over-the-counter sleep remedies?'

'Yes, they do. But we're seeing a decline in sales of Sedix,' the woman says. 'Maybe they aren't running the TV ad any more.'

'What would you recommend?' I ask, explaining that I've had insomnia for sixteen years but that I can no longer take regular sleep medicine.

The technician starts tidying the piles of boxes. 'There isn't any documentation on any of these products,' she says.

I don't understand her answer, but realise I'm going to have to choose for myself and pick up a box of Valerina Forte, simply because its name includes the word *forte*. If I'm going to downgrade from antipsychotics to plants, I may as well opt for the strongest thing on offer.

My last doctor's appointment ended with a referral to a sleep study at Ullenvål Hospital's sleep laboratory. I would have to be extremely patient, the doctor said; the waiting list was long. When I left the doctor's surgery, I felt uplifted: no more pills, a referral had been sent. I would be studied; we would get to the bottom of this.

Sleep laboratory: I picture walking up to the hospital late at night, being met by green-clad doctors and nurses who lay you out on a stretcher and trundle you into a dark room full of enormous machines and measuring devices, place a mask over your nose and mouth, and fasten sensors to your head and chest. And then you're left that way, I imagine, as the doctors and nurses wait on the other side of a huge window for you to fall asleep. In my imagination, several of us bodies lie there that way, lined up on aluminium stretchers and draped in hospital-green sheets like alien abductees. Lying that way, surrounded by millions of kroners' worth of equipment and a medical team on night shift rates waiting around for me to fall asleep sounds like an insomniac's worst nightmare. I'll have to perform sleep to ensure that there will be any sleep for all this expensive monitoring equipment to monitor.

Night. The kids are sleeping, Line is yawning. I'm wide awake. In the pocket of the jacket that hangs in the hallway is the box containing my newly purchased plant-based remedy. I'm not sure whether I want to get Line involved. It's important for me to present the appearance of being a functioning human, especially in her eyes. She knows all about my sleep problems and observes their effects close up. But I can't reveal the entire battle to her: it would be too much for both of us. On the other hand, the latest round of pills gave the whole family a scare and although these are just phony tablets, they are still a substance I'm introducing into my body to achieve a specific effect. A *forte* effect even.

I fetch the box and show it to her. 'It's just herbal, probably won't work. But I thought I ought to try,' I say.

'Valerina,' Line says. 'But you've tried that already.'

'No, I haven't.'

'Yes, you have.'

'When was that?'

'Ages ago. The last time you tried everything.'

The last time I tried everything? Why don't I remember this?

Back when the sleeping pills stopped working, I was still an amateur at lying awake at night. I didn't know it then, but this was just the start of a long career as an insomniac. Without pills to help me, I grew even more desperate. I did everything I now know to be wrong: went to bed earlier in the hope of sleeping longer; stayed in bed the whole night, waiting for sleep to arrive; slept late in the mornings to try and catch up on lost sleep, and did the same thing in the afternoons and at weekends. If I got the chance, I would catch up on the lost sleep to try and get back on an even keel, but then I'd lose my rhythm. The doctor I was seeing in those days could offer no further advice, so I was left to my own devices. And I did what everybody who can't sleep does when the pills stop working and they become desperate enough: I changed my diet; I cut out coffee. I tried first drinking more alcohol, then less and in the end none at all. For several months, I lived an entirely teetotal life and spent Friday nights with my circle of friends drinking lemonade and alcohol-free beer, holding out until the gulf between drunkenness and sobriety became too wide, at which point I would go home. I tried meditation: I went to the ACEM school of meditation on Sporveisgata and took a basic course, where I was given a meditation sound that I repeated to myself as I sat in a swivel chair in the living room. I tried to meditate morning and night, ensuring before each session that Line was either out or in bed. I was afraid she'd die laughing if she saw me sitting there in lotus position, palms turned upward and eyes shut. I almost never manage to free myself from my own gaze, I always see myself from the outside. As I sat there trying to achieve some state or another, I never, for a single second, managed to rid myself of a voice – my own – which said:

Idiot.

Insomnia is also about self-consciousness. A sleepless brain is a brain incapable of ceasing to think about itself. The desire to gain control over sleep can lead to the very opposite. This doesn't just apply to sleep, either. It's like somebody telling you not to think about strawberry ice cream. Of course, you'll think about strawberry ice cream. The American professor of psychology, Daniel Wegner, dealt with this in his theory of *ironic processes of mental control*. He conducted an experiment with 110 students, whom he sent home with a Walkman and a cassette – this was in the eighties – which they were supposed to listen to after going to bed and turning out the light. Half of them heard a message telling them to fall asleep as quickly as possible, while the other half were told to fall asleep whenever they felt like it. The first group slept worst, of course, but it didn't stop there, because that group was also split in two. One part of the group was played stress-inducing marching music and the other, soothing new-age music. The aim was to further increase the stress of subjects who were already stressed about sleeping. And it worked: those who were told to go to sleep rapidly and also heard marching music slept most poorly. What's more, they slept more poorly the whole of that night, long after the music was over. The experiment hadn't just disrupted the process of falling asleep; it had also set in motion the vicious circle of insomnia.[9] The more you think about sleep, the greater your desire for sleep, the smaller the chance that you will sleep. Psychiatry professor Viktor Frankl wrote that sleep is like a 'dove which has landed near one's hand and stays there as long as one does not pay attention to it; if one tries to grab it, it quickly flies away.'[10] This image is akin to my own idea: that sleep is like a stubborn cat I try to coax up onto my lap. The cat only comes when I stop worrying about whether it will. It pads around me on noiseless paws, head lowered, testing me out, waiting and sniffing the air as if it can smell my desperation. I try to forget the cat so that it will leap up onto my lap soundlessly, curl up and fall asleep.

To have insomnia is to be obsessed by the dove or the cat. You haven't slept for several nights and you need sleep: tomorrow morning you have an important meeting scheduled, or you're meeting the girl you like, or you're due to sit an exam, or you're going on a long journey – *everything* depends on being able to sleep. Desperation gains the upper hand. The dove flies off, the cat pads away.

Normal people know they will sleep at night. They expect it. But it isn't a conscious thought. Sleep simply comes, the way it always does. We might compare being able to sleep with a physical task – making a bird table, painting a wall or preparing a meal, say. If we manage to forget ourselves and all our baggage, just disappear into the work, our chances of success are greater. But if we don't manage to forget the self during our work, if we are weighed down by all our cares and thoughts and constantly watch the clock as it ticks its way forward, second by second – then the making or painting or cooking will seem like an insuperable task. My relationship to sleep is very much like my relationship to writing. The more aware I am of sitting and writing, the more difficult it is. The quality of both writing and sleep also diminishes the further I am away from the unconscious. The harder I try, the more difficult it is to achieve. And the more you feel that you need it, the smaller your chances are of getting it. Or as the American comic W. C. Fields put it: 'The best cure for insomnia is to get a lot of sleep.'

No matter how long I sat there in an armchair in a flat in Tøyen all those years ago repeating my meditation sound, no matter how long I *tried*, I never escaped my own self-consciousness. I achieved nothing; on the contrary: the longer I sat, the more I hated myself. Nor did I sleep any better at night.

What else did I try? I went to a psychiatrist who specialised in sleep problems and whose treatment methods included hypnosis. Every Wednesday afternoon I would take the train out to Sandvika, always arriving half an hour early, then stood and waited outside the building where the psychiatrist had his office. He was a short, soft-spoken man with a nervous manner and a small office where we sat facing one another for forty-five minutes. By the time I arrived for the second appointment, he had read all the books I had published to date, and I remember thinking that now it wouldn't be all that easy to back out. He gave me a test consisting of more than a hundred questions and, after looking at my answers, he asked:

'Have you considered the possibility that you might be depressed?'

'No,' I said.

My sleep problems were a mystery to me, but a self-contained mystery, which I didn't link to anything else. I quickly dismissed the thought. Depressed? I just couldn't sleep.

The hypnosis involved closing my eyes as he spoke to me. In this case, too, I was unable to free myself from myself, from that gaze from the outside, but it worked a bit better than the meditation. I always left the psychiatrist's office with a confused sense of having dropped out for a moment, dozed off. He was interested in my dreams and although, as life has gone on, I have had less and less time for the interpretation of dreams, he had a way of placing what I told him about my dreams in the context of what I told him about my life. If I spoke about a dream in which I tried to fight my way through a house full to overflowing with water, as stuffed toys, lampshades and shoes floated by, he would say: 'The house is you. The water is your unconscious.'

Dreams are any mental activity that occurs as we sleep, but most people associate dream activity with the rich experiences of REM sleep.[11] In this stage, certain regions of the brain become far more active: the regions furthest back in the brain that help us to see and form mental images, the part of the cerebral cortex that produces movement, the regions that deal with autobiographical memory, as well as the emotional centres that help create and deal with our feelings. In other words, everything we need to produce emotionally charged action-packed films with ourselves in the starring role. At the same time, the regions that manage rational thought are deactivated. For as long as I have had a conscious relationship to dreams, I have thought of them as the loose ends of the day's impressions. I go through the day and what happens to me is processed in my dreams when I sleep at night. Dreams are films we make using the offcuts on the floor of our mental cutting room once the day is done, or so I've thought. Freud called it the *residue of the day*.

But this turns out not to be strictly true. Studies in which participants wrote down a detailed account of everything they had done during the day and what they dreamt about at night showed that only 1–2 per cent of the dream experiences were repetitions of actual events. But when researchers looked at the emotions people had experienced during the day – anger, grief, joy – they found that 35–55 per cent of the emotional experiences returned in the dreams.[12] Dreams do not recreate events but the feelings that were aroused in us when they happened.

Emotions are also central to sleep scientists' efforts to discover the purpose of dreams. British sleep scientist Matthew Walker believes dreams help us to process and deal with the strong emotions we have experienced during the day to ensure, among other things, that we will later be able to return to past events without being overwhelmed by the emotions originally associated with them. Today, I can think back to a fight I had in Year 7 without having to endure the fear, humiliation and rage I experienced then and there. Walker believes this is the benefit of dreams. And this is what people with post-traumatic stress disorder are unable to achieve. They are incapable of processing, suppressing and ridding themselves of the powerful and unpleasant emotions they once experienced. This is in part because people with this disorder tend to suffer disturbed sleep. Walker thinks that the patients' abnormally high levels of noradrenaline are what prevent healthy dream sleep. They end up in a vicious circle: the mental stress prevents sleep, which could have processed and perhaps eliminated the mental stress. Walker calls it a broken record, because the patients relive the same nightmare night after night without getting better. In experiments[13] that reduced the level of noradrenaline with the aid of medicine, space was created for healthier REM sleep and the nightmares diminished.

Walker has found another advantage of dream sleep:

it fine-tunes our ability to interpret emotions.[14] Walker showed pictures of faces with different emotional expressions to some participants who had slept and some who had not and discovered a remarkable difference. Those who hadn't had their dose of REM sleep were unable to distinguish between one emotion and another. Dream sleep – if not the dreams in themselves – helps us to fine-tune our system for seeing, reading and understanding other people's emotions. Was this the fundamental ability that prolonged, continuous sleep brought with it, setting us apart from other species some time over the course of our evolution – the ability to be a human among humans?

The interpretation of dreams in the psychiatrist's little office in Sandvika led to no improvements in my nightly sleep, and after six months I had to go through the painful process of discontinuing the treatment. He seemed genuinely hurt and surprised when I said it was over. I used the psychiatrist-patient version of *It isn't you, it's me* and blamed it on the long journey.

I contacted a cognitive therapist who specialised in sleep problems. When I rang and explained my situation, he interrupted me midway through my litany of woes. Weirdly, he switched to Bergen-tinged English, although I remember not reacting to that at the time: *You've come to the right place,* he said. The tears welled up, jubilation bubbled in my breast: I had come to the right place. Soon I would be cured!

Cognitive therapy was expensive, and I didn't have a referral from my doctor. I'd reached the point where I no longer dared ask for referrals for further treatment options – and that meant the costs were not covered as they had been with the psychiatrist. But I was so convinced that I didn't care about the money.

The first appointment started with the therapist speaking positively about failing to sleep at night.

'Think of all those free hours! You're a writer, after all – you can write books while the rest of us have to sleep!'

Then he gave me a notepad and a pen.

'I want you to go home and write a list of everything that's stupid about not being able to sleep at night. But also a list of everything that's great. And then I want you to start writing down how you sleep.'

'How I sleep?' I said. 'But I don't sleep. That's why I'm here.'

'So, write that down, then. When you went to bed, when you got up. And then I want you to write down how your days are. Give them star ratings!'

The therapist was a tall thin man with glasses. He sat in the chair opposite me – relaxed, legs crossed, one foot jiggling. Everything about this person exuded balance and energy. What did this guy know about not being able to sleep?

I went home and did my homework, not because I believed in his method but because it would be a total waste of money not to. After two consultations, I dropped out.

With every new offer, every new method, every new person with an approach to my sleep problems I experienced the same internal shift. Wild hope followed by disappointment.

In the end, once I was convinced that all other attempts to get any sleep had been exhausted, Line and I moved out of the city to an old house in the Nordmarka forest: a dry toilet, no running water. Although my hope of getting a good night's sleep was not the sole reason for our move, it was part of that mental balance sheet you draw up every time you change address. Out there it was quiet, with nothing but dogs and chainsaws and forest.

I slept just as poorly, of course I did. And I gave up, partly because I didn't know what else I could come up with to get some sleep, but also because I was starting to accept that my sleep problems were here to stay. The quest was over. After four years, we moved back into the city.

Two years on, here I am again, on a quest to find a cure.

II

I take three tablets of Valerina at ten o'clock, lie watching TV until one, then I go down to my bed, where I fall asleep and wake up half an hour later. It's almost three o'clock before I go back up to the sofa and continue watching the film I interrupted. Only then does it occur to me that we're due at a dinner party the next day.

Is that why I can't get to sleep now?

It's always my first thought every time I make an arrangement that implies some kind of social performance. Being attentive, charming and interesting. What if I don't sleep the night before? It's an *absolute certainty* that I'll be sleep-deprived, that I'll sit there like a shadow of myself. And my friends who know me as garrulous and funny will see me as dull and withdrawn. And worse still, strangers who don't know me will think that this zombie is who I am. This anxiety about not performing socially, not ingratiating myself with everybody I encounter – whether old friends or people I'm meeting for the first time – is something I've had all my life. It's one of the worst aspects of sleeplessness: the strain of having to adapt to others. I can't remember the last time I arrived rested at a party or a night out with friends. If I cancel, I hate myself and my weakness. I generally end up going. Paracetamol, a shot, I almost always manage to pull myself together enough to ensure that nobody notices anything. For a few hours at least.

Sometimes, like now, I'll have forgotten I'm supposed to be doing something important the next day. Only late into the night do I realise why I'm lying awake: I am, of course, due at that party tomorrow; *that's* why I can't sleep. I may forget it, but my insomnia remembers.

I sleep at dawn but am woken shortly afterwards by the boy's first whimperings. I go into his room, then we go upstairs and I switch on the TV. His nappy needs changing and he's hungry. The mornings are always the worst, especially at the weekends. The day feels like a chore, and an endless one at that. We're supposed to spend the whole day together and I have so little to give.

Line gets up at nine and I can go back down to the bedroom and try again. I lie on my bed and put on the *White Album*, which is long enough if I should happen to fall asleep. The bedclothes are clean, the duvet is cold and airy, the bedroom is quiet and cool. The feeling of lying in your own bed, a mattress supporting your body: just soft enough, just firm enough. The darkness that enfolds me, the weight of the duvet against my skin, my naked feet rubbing against one another in sheer well-being, the pillow around my ears, the warmth filling me from within, my eyes unable to stay open —

That feeling does not come. Instead, the bed rejects me, the way the body rejects a foreign organ. I feel as if I've sneaked into some event uninvited. I roll over onto my side. *You know I can't sleep, I can't stop my brain*, sings

39

John Lennon. I draw my feet up beneath me. I adjust my pillow. I roll over onto my back again. *I'll give you everything I've got for a little peace of mind.*

No.

This isn't working.

'Did you manage to get any sleep?' Line asks when I go upstairs again three-quarters of an hour later.

'A bit,' I say and smile.

I make myself a cup of coffee. My insomnia, which means I have to be extra careful with the timing and amounts of caffeine I consume, has probably further reinforced my love of coffee. What's more, I continually have to defend my coffee-drinking to Line, who thinks that if I really want to sleep better, cutting out coffee will be a small price to pay. She's right of course. Even so, I carry on. It must be frustrating for her to have to deal with a person who wipes away his tears over being unable to sleep at night with one hand while holding an enormous mug of extra-strong coffee in the other. Line shoulders a significant share of the burden of my sleeplessness; I'm bound to listen to her. So several times I've stopped drinking coffee for long periods: one week, two weeks, three weeks without coffee. I've never detected any major difference in my sleeping problems and then, slowly but surely, I resume my coffee drinking.

I drink the first cup and make myself another. I'm feeling sorry for myself, and besides I have to keep awake for the party tonight, not for my own sake but for Line's, I think in self-justification, as I grind the beans in the coffee-mill, making such a racket that everybody in the house can hear what I'm up to. After a few minutes the pot starts to gurgle and steam. After the second dose, it's as if my heart steps up its tempo in my chest. Caffeine is a reviving and stimulating substance. It can bind itself to the same place as adenosine, which is the substance that makes us wearier the longer we stay awake. Caffeine sneaks into the same receptors in the brain and blocks the adenosine, so that it doesn't get a chance to work[15]. That way we avoid feeling tired.

Seven out of ten Norwegians drink coffee daily. On average, we drink 3.7 cups a day. And the consumption is steady. In Norway, we drink roughly as much coffee today as we did twenty years ago.[16] The big question when it comes to coffee and sleep is, of course: when in the day should you stop drinking coffee in order to sleep at night?

The idea that caffeine intake during the day can keep you awake at night is not some hysterical claim. Skipping that afternoon coffee can actually help you sleep better. A normal cup of coffee contains roughly 120 milligrams of caffeine. If you're used to a lot of coffee, you'll need more to wake up. As long as we have a certain amount of caffeine in our system, we'll notice the changes. The caffeine level in the body is at its highest around half an hour after the coffee is drunk. In addition, when coffee is broken down in the liver, it is split into three substances, all of which have an invigorating effect. Finally, the caffeine has a diuretic effect. But caffeine hangs around in the body long after the tangible effect has abated. The average half-life of caffeine – in other words, the time it takes to break the dose down to half – is five hours. My two strong cups of coffee – roughly 240 milligrams of caffeine – were drunk at midday and will be reduced to 120 milligrams by five o'clock in the afternoon. By ten o'clock at night, the level will have fallen to around 60 milligrams. At some point, and long before I'll be heading home for bed, the amount of caffeine will be so tiny that it will no longer have any invigorating effect.

At the dinner party, I sit beside a couple I haven't met before. He talks about taking executives on hunting trips in the Norwegian mountains to shoot ptarmigan and deer. She does some kind of humanitarian work. It's a relief, I notice, to be here at last, to be up and running. It's going better than I'd feared. And in a few hours, it'll be over.

Then it's my turn. I tell them that I work as a speech-writer and author.

'An author! What do you write about?' she asks.

'Right now, I'm thinking of writing about my own sleeplessness. I've had insomnia for many years.'

Where did that come from? And why now? Is it because my days are so full of my quest for a solution that it's all spilling over? I'm not in the habit of introducing myself as an insomniac at parties. *Hi, my name is Anders and I can't sleep.*

'How interesting!' she says. 'I sleep badly too.'

'Is that so?' I'm both confused and fired up, not just because of meeting another person with sleep problems but also because I have revealed my own.

'I wake up at seven in the morning, even at weekends. I usually drink some milk,' she says. 'Then I fall asleep again.'

'You should go hunting,' he says. 'That'll make you sleep, I guarantee it.'

Soon the whole table is talking about sleep problems. I don't know if it's because they see me as somebody with a history of suffering whom they feel obliged to listen to or whether it's because they all consider themselves experts on their own nightly sleep. The host tells us about a bad night two weeks earlier. Another person has a son who's turned his cycle on its head, staying up all night and sleeping all day. Somebody says I must try acupuncture – it works. Another promises to send me a link for American herbal teas.

'You have to cut out flour and sugar,' the hostess says.

'Have you done a sleep study?'

'What colour are your bedroom walls? Not yellow, I hope.'

'You must borrow my cabin – I always sleep so soundly there.'

'Masturbation,' the woman beside me whispers in my ear. 'That makes me sleep like a baby.'

On our way home at two o'clock, I take the three Valerina tablets I've brought with me in my rucksack. I get into bed and fall asleep quickly, thanks either to the wine or the Valerina or my own natural ability to doze off – I don't much care as long as I go to sleep. When I wake at four, however, the investigation is opened. Is it the wine that woke me? Is it the alcohol on its way out of my system? Did I take enough Valerina tablets? And that coffee – how much did I actually drink and how long ago was it now? I lie there thinking of all the sleep advice that was offered around the table. Family and friends also tend to proffer tips whenever I complain about sleep. This advice, I've noticed, is more likely to give me an insight into the person giving the advice than into my problem. It is always well intentioned, but it isn't based on knowledge: the person giving the advice is basing it on what works best for them. Even so, I know I'll store these tips away and even – when I get desperate enough – try some of them out. Who knows, maybe the cure for sleeplessness really is to lie in a hunting cabin, wanking and drinking milk.

If you get little enough sleep, anything can start sounding sensible in the end.

III

Monday. Nothing but bills in the mailbox. I'm still waiting for the letter from Ullevål Hospital; it's been over a month since the referral was sent. I send an electronic message to my doctor via the surgery website. The letter that should have come a long time ago hasn't arrived – what's going on? On Tuesday, I sign up for a course of yoga to improve sleep and book an appointment for acupuncture treatment focused on sleep disorders. I also Google *sleep* and *chiropractic*, but don't find any offers of treatment, only theory. On Wednesday, I buy two new books about sleep: Arianna Huffington's *The Sleep Revolution* and Shawn Stevenson's *Sleep Smarter*.

So far I have read books on sleep written by doctors and psychologists, most of them Norwegian. It's surprising how little we actually know and how new the knowledge in the field seems to be. And it is disappointing to see how insomnia is marginalised in all the books about sleep and sleep disorders. Often, this one sleep problem, *my* problem, gets fobbed off with a two-page sub-chapter alongside all the other sleep problems. It's the same with Arianna Huffington's book, which I abandon before getting even halfway through. All it does is make me angry. Her introduction to the topic of sleep goes like this: she has lived her life as a successful businesswoman, but it has come at a price. She opted out of sleep in order to follow her dream. Some years ago, she had a breakdown caused by sleep deprivation and now she lives a new and better life in which she spends more time sleeping. We're in the middle of a sleep crisis, Huffington has realised. Opting out of sleep in favour of job and career is life-threatening. The most provoking aspect of the book is the way Huffington illustrates the problem: anecdote after anecdote about successful and generally famous people (all apparently friends of the author, since she is on first-name terms with all of them: Brad, Jennifer, Kate) who don't sleep enough because they're too busy being talented and famous.

The second book seems a bit more empathetic, with its promise of *21 Essential Strategies*. Impatiently I flip past the foreword and the introduction until I get to the first tips: 'Start to think of sleep as an incredible indulgence, like a sensuous dessert, a relaxing massage, a hot date with someone special, or something else you really look forward to. *I've got a hot date with sleep tonight, and we are really going to get—it—on!* Start letting go of the stress surrounding sleep and allow yourself to enjoy it. You work hard enough in your life as it is. Treat yourself to some incredible sleep. You deserve it.'[17]

What the hell?

I read through the list of 21 tips. Some of them seem sensible – like getting more sunlight during the day, getting up early and avoiding screen time before bed. Other advice seems vague and far too general, like 'enjoy the benefits that the big "O" can add to your life', 'Create a sleep sanctuary' and 'Know the value of sleep'. Some of the advice is incomprehensible, like the last one: *Get grounded*. 'Make it a regular practice,' writes Stevenson, 'to get some quality time with your bare feet on the ground: This means conductive surfaces like soil, grass, sand (at the beach) and even living bodies of water like the ocean.'[18]

Can't sleep? Try standing around for a while.

I flick through the book looking for details of the author but can't find anything. Who is this person who's supposed to be teaching me to sleep smarter? Who is Shawn Stevenson? Are they a woman or a man, and what do they know about not being able to sleep? I get the same feeling I had with Huffington's book: that it's written for people who *can* sleep if they want to. The book wants to convince readers that sleep is important. I need no convincing. I *know* that sleep deprivation is dangerous. I'd do anything to be able to sleep eight hours a night. It's painful to read about the health risk of sleep deprivation in a book aimed at people for whom sleep is only a matter of willpower; books that simply don't take into account the existence of people like me who lack the *ability* to sleep. The message in both books implies that sleep is just lying there waiting, an abundance of it – all you need to do is help yourself. Because you're worth it.

Now I understand how it must feel for people with anorexia to read diet tips. *There's so much good and nourishing food. Pull yourself together, eat!*

I put the books aside. On the following nights, I increase the Valerina dose to four and five tablets, but I feel nothing, so I give up – I can't be bothered to take them for two weeks to achieve the *optimal effect*, as it says on the packet. In the nights that follow, I notice no difference; I sleep no more poorly.

IV

My prejudices against yoga are confirmed at the *Yoga for better sleep* course:

    I'm the only male participant

    They serve herbal tea

Crazy, undocumented claims about what happens in the brain and body.

I thought all it took to do yoga was a body and an exercise mat, but yoga people turn out to be equipment freaks too, just like the rest of us. Every participant is handed two mats, a blanket, two large bolsters, two support blocks, two smaller bolsters, a bag to place over themselves and a smaller bag to place over their face. The course leader, a small, nimble woman, recommends various sleep apps and offers advice about how to use headphones in bed without getting too tangled up in the wires. The course starts at 6.30 p.m. on a Friday evening and lasts three hours, which means I have to leave home just before Line puts the kids to bed. So far, my efforts to find something to help me sleep have been pursued during the day and they have generally been completed within three-quarters of an hour. Now it's a three-hour course on a Friday evening. What next? A weekend seminar at a mountain hotel? My efforts to relieve stress have left me more stressed than ever before. So far Line has been patient, but I sense that I am approaching the limits.

It was my friend Liv who told me about the course; she took it ten years ago when she was pregnant with her second child and couldn't sleep. She is sleeping poorly again, she says: she wakes in the middle of the night, then lies there brooding. She has come along with me and I'm happy not to be alone. First there are those not-so-welcoming e-mail admonitions that, in brief, instruct us to arrive punctually, soundlessly and odourlessly. Then there's the panic when I realise that I'm the only man, a terror that is exacerbated by the course leader, who – as she tells everybody to settle on their mats for introductory relaxation – places a blanket over me and *nobody else*. This special treatment does not aid relaxation. Fortunately, Liv is lying on the mat next to mine. We're barely able even to whisper to one another, so subdued is the atmosphere at the centre.

'What do we do if we have to laugh?' Liv says.

Then we lie there with cushions beneath our necks and ankles – lights dimmed, soothing music barely audible, the course leader's voice gentle and friendly – and I find that I am lying comfortably. Despite all the equipment and the complicated philosophy, yoga boils down to finding a comfortable position.

We are treated to a long introduction about how yogic philosophy, also known as *ayurveda*, perceives sleep. There are three different types of sleeping pattern: *vata*, *pitta* and *kapha*. Some of the advice sounds sensible. For example: we sit crouched in front of a screen all day, in a position that signals stress and fear. That's why it's important to straighten up and stretch, to bring body and mind into balance. Okay, I think. I do sit like that throughout my working day. I have developed a somewhat stooped posture. And my sleep problems arrived at the same time as I started working. I should at least check this out. Straightening up and stretching now and again can't do any harm.

But when the course leader starts talking about circadian rhythm, she totally loses me with the claims she makes: that the body switches from liver power to lung power at three o'clock every morning – then it's lung time, she says; or that the pineal gland, the region of the brain that releases melatonin, expands through meditation, and that people who have meditated a great deal over their lifetime have been found to have *enormous* pineal glands. She makes a circle with a thumb and forefinger. In the end, the course leader and one of the participants start to discuss how much daylight can pass through glasses and contact lenses – or whether people who rely on optical aids are doomed to a life without circadian rhythm.

I don't believe a few millimetres of glass can disrupt a rhythm so fundamental to all living creatures on Earth.

A cell group in the middle of the brain known as the *nucleus suprachiasmaticus* serves as a twenty-four-hour clock for humans and all other living species.[19] Humanity's internal clock is not as accurately set as one might think. There are roughly twenty-four hours and fifteen minutes in a day and night, so we have to adjust ourselves by a quarter of an hour in every daily cycle. This is part of the reason why it is easier to fly west than east. The jetlag isn't so bad because our body is already adjusted for a bit of extra time.

In order to adjust we need the external clock, the sun. Or its proxy, electric light. When light strikes the eye, signals travel to the *nucleus suprachiasmaticus*, which is responsible for activating the parts of the brain that wake us up and deactivating the parts that make us tired. Our brightly lit, white-tiled bathrooms may be practical for performing the last routines of our day, but they are a direct assault on the sleep for which we are preparing. That is also why you should avoid switching on the bathroom light when you get up in the night to pee: it tricks the brain into thinking that the day has begun.

When the light vanishes, this process will be reversed and the processes that make us tired, such as melatonin production, start up.[20] Melatonin is sent out into the blood from the pineal gland – which is the size of a corn kernel – and serves as a messenger: it's getting dark. It'll soon be time for sleep! Melatonin isn't sleep-inducing in itself but it helps *set in motion* the processes the brain undergoes in order to sleep. So melatonin production is a prelude to actually going to sleep: during the night and towards daybreak, production slows. Its job is done. In the evening and towards the night, it increases again: the melatonin signals new sleep.

French chronobiologist Jean-Jacques D'Ourtous de Mairan was the first person to prove that living creatures have evolved an inbuilt circadian rhythm, in 1729. He did this by placing a flower, a heliotrope, in a room whose lighting was constant day and night; he saw that the leaves continued to open and close in the same way they did when they were exposed to sunlight and dark of night.[21] The switch between an active and inactive state continued even though the assumed cause – the sun – was eliminated. Nearly three hundred years later, in 2017, three Americans won the Nobel Prize in Medicine for identifying a protein in the cells of fruit flies that increased at night and decreased by day. They had located the workings of the clock that ticked inside all living beings – workings imprinted on our very genetic material by the passage of the sun millions, maybe billions of years ago, and to which life has adapted.

All living beings need rest, but not all of them follow the sun. There are exceptions. In dark caves beneath the desert of Somalia lives a blind fish with an unusually long circadian rhythm: 43 hours. Bees have a kind of social inner clock that is capable of 'switching off' its own circadian rhythm, enabling them to tend to the colony's young without a break. Migratory birds are also able to suspend their circadian rhythm and go without sleep for long periods – sometimes several weeks – until they have reached their goal. It's far from easy for animals living in Polar regions to follow the sun. Norwegian scientists who monitored reindeer both on Svalbard and in Finnmark, northern Norway, discovered that the animals simply didn't have a circadian rhythm for large parts of the year.[22]

As a species, we are not homogeneous in our circadian rhythm. The notion of early birds and night owls isn't a myth. Roughly 40 per cent of the world's population wakes at around sunrise and functions best in the morning. Some 30 per cent generally go to sleep later and wake later in the morning. The last 30 per cent fall into an intermediate category. The difference lies in the prefrontal cortex and is genetic. When a night owl is 'forced' to get up, their prefrontal cortex is still switched off and doesn't begin working properly until later in the day.[23] If we take into account evolution and humanity in its state of nature, it seems logical that both human types should exist. If people sleep at different times, there will be a longer period in which part of the herd is awake, and this makes the community less vulnerable to external threats. In a modern, conformist society where most people sleep behind locked doors, this division no longer has a function. Society has chosen, and the winners were early birds (or *vata* people, if we are to stick to Ayurvedic philosophy).

When you sleep and when you wake doesn't just depend on your inbuilt circadian rhythm, but also on how long you have been awake. This is one of humanity's most fundamental flaws: the longer we are awake, the wearier we become. This is called sleep pressure and is caused by a substance called adenosine – the same substance that caffeine blocks. If you've just slept, you don't have much adenosine. If it's a long time since you slept, you have a lot of it. The concentration of adenosine increases over the course of the day and when we sleep at night, it is eliminated, preparing us for a new day.

Circadian rhythm and sleep pressure – and the inter-action between them – are factors that we relate to every day and night. If we look at the curves described by these two processes, circadian rhythm and sleep pressure are furthest away from one another at night. We get tired and want to sleep. If we don't go to bed, the curves will start to approach one another and many people will find themselves livening up. The sleep pressure is still there, because we haven't slept, but the circadian rhythm persists regardless of our actions. In the morning, the two curves meet and make us wakeful. By the afternoon, they are far apart again and we are sleepy once more.

If we do anything that disrupts the natural progression of these curves, we may have problems. If we treat ourselves to a three-hour nap after dinner it isn't so easy to fall asleep at the normal time, no matter how good our inbuilt circadian rhythm is. That is because we have depleted the sleep pressure that had built up. If we have been up late at night, it may be more difficult to get the much-needed eight hours of sleep; instead of sleeping late into the day, most people find that their circadian rhythm kicks in: we wake up in the morning and can't sleep any more, even though the sleep pressure is still there.

These forces that control our sleep are the result of a rhythm that originated at the same time as the stars and the planets. Fourteen billion years ago, the universe came into being. Our star, the sun, was created ten billion years later, at the same time as our own planet. The Earth rotates on its axis, which causes the light of the sun to come and go on every point of the planet's surface (except the Polar regions). When life came about roughly 3.8 billion years ago, it adapted to these conditions. Just as life optimises oxygen intake in the blood according to the oxygen content of the atmosphere, it also aligns its rest with the sun's passage across the sky. It grows light, it grows dark, and it grows light again. Sleep finds its place in the absence of the sun, in the darkness and cold; and it grows, becomes longer and more continuous and, as a result, deeper. Our forebears made their way into trees and caves, not just to protect themselves from predators and the cold and storms, but also to rest. To be able to sleep. For billions of years life rises and sets with the sun – until at last the circadian rhythm runs independently: it is *within us*, deep in the genes of every living being – right up until the day when a specimen of the increasingly self-obsessed and self-contradictory human species finds himself lying on a yoga mat in Oslo, legs up the wall, supported by five bolsters and thinking:

Why can't I get to sleep?

JUNE

Night and Day

About sleep deprivation and what it does to rats and philosophers; about heartbreak and other mental affliction; and the story of the music teacher who died from lack of sleep.

I

The night of Monday 13th June: I went to bed at 11 p.m., switched the light off at 11.30 p.m. Lay awake for twenty minutes, got up again. Slept on the sofa some time before 12.30 a.m. and didn't wake until 6.45 a.m., when the boy woke up. Last night's sleep: deep. Daytime functioning: very good.

I've started keeping a sleep journal, the way I tried to when I was seeing that wildly expensive cognitive therapist a few years back and the way the sleep scientist Bjørn Bjorvatn recommends in his book, *Better Sleep*. 'Many people who are struggling with sleep difficulties become more conscious of the nature of their sleep difficulty if they keep a sleep journal,' writes Bjorvatn. But like all the measures I take to deal with my sleep difficulties – it appears superfluous after a couple of hours' sleep. Why the journal? I'm sleeping, aren't I? It's the same with the acupuncture appointment I made – I don't need it now. And as for the referral my doctor sent to Ullevål Hospital, two months have now gone by without any news of the sleep study. Maybe it's just as well?

Everybody in the family has had enough sleep this morning, so the routines work. I get the kids out into the bike trailer and cycle off through the entranceway at 7.40 a.m. I drop both the kids off, and even manage to make them laugh before we part ways. It isn't even eight o'clock yet when I lock the bike and trailer outside the Business School and go inside, buy myself a coffee and sit down with my Mac and sandwiches. Within minutes, I'm engrossed in the manuscript I'm working on. An hour later, it's as though I emerge from a trance. Two pages of text have been filled. I close my Mac and cycle the hundred metres over to the ministry. I eat a slice of bread as I go through the security gates, pick up a cup of coffee on my way into the office, log on and let the computer pull itself together as I get myself ready. When I've slept, I'm an efficient person, capable of getting the three basic functions – clothes, breakfast, toilet break – out of the way so that I can make a start on actual production. If I'm going to get anything done, I have to prioritise. Some days I don't even tie my shoelaces before lunch.

I complete a speech I started the day before and send it to the technical department for quality assurance. Over the course of the morning, two new tasks come in. I cancel the acupuncture appointment. I call Line and we agree to go to Ålesund and visit my family in autumn. Then I send a message to Mum.

Lunch. Ten minutes late, I run across to the bakery by the river. Andreas is sitting there with a coffee and some notes in front of him. I apologise, buy myself a coffee and we start exchanging ideas. Andreas and I have a cartoon that runs in *Klassekampen* newspaper every day. Andreas turns up with a list of ideas but my page is blank; I haven't managed to think about this in advance – I get most of my ideas on the spot. Since the summer holidays are approaching, we have to deliver six weeks' worth of strips before we can take a break.

'Can you deliver the text for eighteen strips tomorrow?' Andreas asks before we part.

'Will twelve do? I can send the rest later.'

'Fine.'

At four o'clock, I pick up the kids and cycle home. Before dinner, I get two new drafts of the minister's opinion piece sent off. We eat and I do the washing-up. As the kids watch TV, I sit down beside them and pull out my mobile phone. First I order some photo frames. Then I make a start on the text for the cartoon strips and get the first six sent off before it's time to put the kids to bed. Supper, a wash, nightclothes, toothbrushing. As I wait for the girl to fall asleep, I sit beside her bed with my laptop, going through a draft of an opinion piece. Soon I hear her breathing deeply. I go upstairs, clear up and put on the dishwasher. As the machine starts churning away, a melody attaches itself to the regular rhythm. Before I can forget it, I pull out my mobile phone and sing the melody line into it.

I go back to the living room and see that Line has fallen asleep in front of the TV. I wake her up. For a moment she is confused, then she stretches and yawns.

'I dropped off.'

'You should go down to bed and get a proper night's sleep,' I say.

Line goes to bed.

Outside, the string of lights and the two lanterns we hung up in the big pear tree start to shine in the dusk. On the lawn are two red mini-goals, a handful of balls and the remnants of a badminton net. The white garden table glows in the summer darkness. It'll soon be midnight and even now the sky is pale grey behind the fruit trees and the houses. A new day is on its way before the old one is over.

I have the flat and the next few hours to myself. I sit at the writing desk, open up my Mac and place my guitar on my knee.

I can see why a lot of people have a romantic perception of what it means to be sleepless: the insomniac with a glass of wine and a jazz album on in the background. Leonard Cohen once said: 'The last refuge of the insomniac is a sense of superiority to the sleeping world.' Line has touched on this a number of times. *Sometimes I think you want to be up at night.* And yes, it does have its advantages. If you eliminate sleep deprivation from the equation, you get more time; and that's not all: you have the world to yourself and time for the big thoughts. Everybody else is sleeping. At night, everything seems amplified – existence no longer stares you in the eye but takes a step back. A space opens up where you can observe and think.

Over the ages, philosophers have shunned sleep and embraced sleeplessness. For most thinkers, the constant consciousness and restlessness of insomnia must seem the ideal state for insight, whereas sleep is unconsciousness, and the absence of thought and pondering. Plato said: 'When a man is asleep, he is no better than if he were dead; and he who loves life and wisdom will take no more sleep than is necessary for health.' Five hundred years later, the theologian Clement of Alexandria said there was no more use in a sleeping man than a dead man. 'The owl of Minerva spreads its wings only with the falling of the dusk,' wrote Hegel in the 1700s. Nietzsche believed that the goal of all good Europeans should be wakefulness. In his book *In Praise of Insomnia*, from 1976, the philosopher Emmanuel Lévinas wrote that sleeplessness was the very epicentre of insight, while another philosopher and psychoanalyst, Anne Dufourmantelle, put it this way: 'Philosophy was born with anxiety, with questioning, with insomnia. It takes upon itself the ills of the world, and thus it cannot sleep.' A good philosopher is a sleepless philosopher. The only one who seems to break away from the tradition of philosophical history is Descartes, who viewed sleep as something a great thinker must be sure to get enough of. 'Sleep is nourishment for the brain,'[24] he wrote. Descartes used to make sure he got twelve hours' sleep – from midnight until midday – every night. When he moved to Sweden to work for the Swedish queen, he was forced to get up early in the morning and died of pneumonia shortly afterwards.

When I eventually come to myself again and look at the clock, it is quarter to one. Making music is an obsession incompatible with sleep: my heart beats faster, I am uplifted and cannot come down. I must be careful, I thought, I must calm myself. I put down my guitar and close my Mac.

Night of Tuesday 14th June: lay down on the sofa at 1 a.m., fell asleep in front of the TV at around 2 a.m. Woke up at 5.30 a.m., went to bed but couldn't sleep any more. Got up at 6.45 a.m. Last night's sleep: deep. Daytime functioning: great.

Three-and-a-half hours' decent sleep, maybe four – that's all I need. I feel replenished, ready for a new day. I leave for work early and walk up to the kindergarten, where they're having a summer party. We eat hotdogs, I talk to the other parents and the kindergarten staff.

Without sleep, I would have struggled with words, doubt restraining my every sentence. But today, I stand in the middle of the crowd and chat with semi strangers about standing in queues with kids, about moving to Røa, about going on holiday to Koster, about how brilliant the kindergarten staff are.

Line puts the kids to bed as I get on my bike and cycle west through the city to a music studio in Smestad, where Kåre and I meet once a week to record music. We keep at it, laying down vocals and guitars and drums until it's time to spare a thought for the neighbours.

I cycle home and in the silent flat I hear the echo of the music and my own pulse beating in my ears. The others are asleep. First I wash up and clean the kitchen, then I open up my Mac and carry on where I left off the night before, on one of my own musical projects. When it gets to one o'clock, I pack it in. I don't want to – I feel wide awake – but I have to try and settle for the night. TV on, I lie down on the sofa with my mobile and swipe through internet news sites and e-mails. The last thing I do before putting down my phone is write the text for six new comic strips and send them to Andreas. Then I check my mail, even though I shouldn't do that right before bedtime. Part of me is crackling, wants more, doesn't want to sleep, wants to carry on through the night, feels so good.

Another part thinks: It's going to blow.

II

Night of Wednesday 15th June. Lay awake on the sofa until 5 a.m. Slept lightly, on and off, for an hour. Then lay awake until the boy woke up at 7 a.m. Got up. Last night's sleep: very light. Daytime functioning: very poor.

The sky is low and pale grey; there are wet patches on the flagstones of the staircase. My feet are ice cold, my neck damp with sweat. My finger joints and back ache. I stand at the kitchen window looking out at the bike, which is padlocked to the stair rail, thinking about everything I have to get done before I can cycle off. I have to undo the padlock, hook up the trailer…

'We'll take the car today,' I say.

On my way out of the kindergarten, a staff member stops me. I try to follow what she's saying – some funny thing my son did at lunch yesterday – but all I'm capable of registering is that she has slept well. Clear eyes, glowing skin, physical vitality, her words flowing swiftly and with ease. She seems to be bubbling over with surplus energy and joy. When I reply, my voice feels muffled with cotton wool and emerges from some place ten centimetres away from my head.

I sit down at my regular spot at the Business School and open my Mac, then sit there gazing into space. Morning-fresh, well-slept young people. I look at the page of text in front of me: dead black symbols.

I'll never make it as a writer.

To get into the department's basement car park I have to pass through several barriers with codes. I can't remember the code until the car behind me beeps, sending me into a panic, and then the numbers seem to tumble out of my fingers.

My stomach rumbles before ten o'clock. I go down to the canteen alone, an hour before the others will eat lunch. At two minutes past ten, I'm sitting in the most secluded corner of the canteen, shovelling down meatloaf and gravy from a plate piled so high that it spills over onto the tray. I spread *Dagbladet* out in front of me on the table; the headline on one of the front-page stories is: 'How to sleep better.'

An SMS ticks in from Mum, asking if I've bought plane tickets for the trip we discussed. I don't reply. Formulating a response, thinking about the trip and all the negotiations with different family members that it will entail seems impossible right now. At the same time, my guilty conscience gnaws at me. I'm such a bad son.

In the afternoon a mail arrives from Andreas, who's chasing the last comic strips. I reply that they're coming. I pick up the children and we get a pizza on the way home. After eating, I lie on the sofa, swiping through online news sites, following one link after another without knowing where they'll lead. My sleep-deprived brain picks out only the quick carbs: whatever is easily understood, cartoonish, compressed; it always follows the path of least resistance then carries steadily onwards without committing to anything whatsoever.

As I wait for the kids to fall asleep, I make a new acupuncture appointment. And a new doctor's appointment. It's time to find out what's happening with that referral.

Night of Thursday 16th June. Go to bed at 10.30 p.m., go to sleep but wake up again at 11.30 p.m. Get up again, lie down on the sofa and watch films until 4.30 a.m. Slept? Awake from around 5.30 a.m. Get up with the children at 6.30 a.m. Last night's sleep: very light. Daytime functioning: very bad.

Over the days that follow, it feels as if a leaden cloak is being draped over me: my body is heavy, my breathing is heavy, my head is heavy, everything is heavy. There's a knot in my midriff, like a sob that is never released. I am capable of working at my normal pace for a few hours in the morning and then it stops dead. I'm unable to do any writing on my own projects. I can't cope with meeting other people. Only during a few brief moments of the day, when I'm with the children and Line, do I feel it lift – small things get through to me, radiate light. I don't turn up for my doctor's appointment; I can't even be bothered to cancel. What good will it do me now? I'm waiting for it to pass. And I'm waiting to get some sleep. If I can only sleep, I'll be myself again.

Night of Friday 17th June. Go to bed at 2 a.m. and get up again at 3 a.m. Fall asleep at 5.30 a.m., wake up at 7 a.m. Last night's sleep: very bad. Daytime functioning: very bad.

Sleeplessness is the very epicentre of insight.

What a load of absolute bollocks.

Philosophers discuss sleep and sleeplessness as abstract concepts. Philosophers confuse insomnia with *absence of sleep*. They don't know what they're talking about. Insomnia is not freedom. It's the opposite: insomnia binds us; it is sleep that liberates. The thinking man is supposed to be alert, conscious, critical, enquiring, inquisitive and restless – but without sleep, humans lose almost *all these qualities*. The insomniac is uncritical, indifferent, lazy, incapable of taking anything in or classifying knowledge. Only the restlessness remains. In order to truly open our eyes, we must first close them.

There is just one philosopher who suffered from insomnia, Emil Cioran of Romania, who does not talk about the condition as an ideal but as an egotistical and physical state. Unsurprisingly, he is one of the most sceptical and pessimistic thinkers in the history of philosophy. He had an above-average interest in suicide. Cioran succumbed to Alzheimer's disease, disappearing into oblivion and confusion before his death. This description of insomnia leaves us in no doubt that he knew what he was talking about. 'You will suffer from everything, and to excess: the winds will seem gales; every touch a dagger; smiles, slaps; trifles, cataclysms.'[25]

Night of Saturday 18th June. Sleep from 5 a.m. to 7 a.m. Last night's sleep: very bad. Daytime functioning: bad.

To lie awake at night is to be captive to the clock; you are obsessed with it. Everything you do, everything you are, is defined by the time of day. It's two o'clock, you can't sleep; it's three o'clock, you can't sleep. At the same time, you are outside time. You can't sleep because your inner clock has stopped. You can *see* that the clock is showing 1.45 a.m., you *know* that the time is 1.45 a.m., but your body doesn't care.

Everybody else sleeps, every night throughout their life. Five hours, six, seven, eight, nine. My children sleep eleven hours every night. If I had been deprived of food in this way over sixteen years, I would look like a walking corpse. My ribs would protrude, my eyes would shine palely in their sockets, my skin would be pulled taut over cheekbones and chin. The people around me would raise the alarm, force-feeding me if necessary.

I do not live, I merely exist, says one of the sleepless patients in Bjørn Bjorvatn's book.

Night of Sunday 19th June. The sofa again. Sleep from 4.30 a.m. to 6 a.m. Last night's sleep: very bad. Daytime functioning: can't cope any more.

III

The medical books I read about sleep are mostly filled with material about *how* we sleep – the different stages of sleep; how the brain and the rest of the body switch mode as we pass from a waking state into sleep. But when I come to the big question, *why* we sleep, there is little of value. I find only phrases worthy of a primary school kid: We sleep to *save energy*. We sleep to *prepare our body for a new day*. In some books, there's even a question mark at the end – we can't even be absolutely certain of this.

There are dozens of theories. One is that sleep is energy saving – that we sleep for a large part of every twenty-four-hour cycle to save calories, simple as that. At first this sounds sensible, but studies have shown that the energy saved by lying still for an entire night is equivalent to the energy obtained from a hotdog.[26] Another theory is that sleep is a kind of workshop, where the body and brain are rebuilt and maintained. A third theory suggests that we sleep to give our brain a chance to process and consolidate everything it has experienced and learned during the day. One theory doesn't rule out the other, but there is no single, unambiguous answer.

What sleep science has managed to agree on in a sense is what happens if we *don't* sleep.

There are also several individual stories and fates that demonstrate the results. In 1959, American radio DJ Peter Tripp went just over eight days without sleep. The stunt was called a 'wakeathon' and could be followed by anybody who was interested – the radio host sat in a glass booth in Times Square, New York. After three days he started to yell at the people around him; after five days, he suffered hallucinations and paranoia. His body temperature dropped. On his last day of wakefulness, Tripp became convinced that his own doctor was an undertaker.

During the European Cup in 2012, Chinese football supporter Jiang Xiaoshan decided to watch all the matches at night while continuing to go to work in the daytime. After eleven days and nights without sleep, he was found dead. England and France were his favourites.[27]

There are also cases of people who have stopped sleeping against their will and have ended up dying of it – like the terrible story of Michael Corke, a music teacher from New Lexon, US.[28] After turning forty Corke started to sleep more and more poorly, until one day he stopped sleeping altogether. He was suffering from a rare genetic disease known as fatal familial insomnia. The thalamus, the filter in the brain that shuts out all sensory impressions when we fall asleep, is perforated by a prion protein. The brain is no longer capable of shutting out the conscious perception of everything that happens around us – the sensory doors are always open. Corke was awake twenty-four hours a day. There was no cure. Week after week, month after month – not a second's sleep. He became like an old man, barely capable of walking. After six months without sleep, Corke was bedbound and dying. He was incapable of looking after himself, lacked language and was beset by endless hallucinations and delusions. 'Should you have observed Corke at this time,' Walker writes, 'it would be clear how desperate he was for sleep. His eyes would make your own feel tired. His blinks were achingly slow as if the eyelids wanted to stay shut, mid-blink, and not reopen for days. They telegraphed the most despairing hunger for sleep you could imagine.' After eight months without sleep, Corke died.

If sleep deprivation is fatal – what do we die of?

An experiment conducted in the 1980s involved keeping rats awake for long periods by placing them on a small, unstable platform above cold water. Over the course of two weeks, the unfortunate creatures developed patches in their fur, wounds that wouldn't heal, and they lost weight regardless of how much they ate. In the end they died.[29] There was no doubt that sleep deprivation was what killed them. But how?

It takes more than one bad night for a person to die of sleep deprivation. Even people like me, who may have severe sleep problems over prolonged periods, are a long way off a deadly outcome. But before death occurs, other aspects of body and mind fail. Temperature, for example. The less sleep, the poorer the control over body temperature. In this respect all mammals, including humans, are vulnerable: our physiological processes can only occur within a small temperature range. If we end up outdoors, we die. Maintaining a good, steady body temperature is the responsibility of a cell group deep in the brain known as the hypothalamus. During sleep, our metabolism slows. In light or deep sleep, our temperature falls; during REM sleep, the hypothalamus stops regulating temperature altogether. A study has shown that sleep deprivation leads to poor co-ordination of the blood circulation in the skin, causing certain parts of the body to become colder – especially the hands and feet.[30] The experiment with the rats showed that, when deprived of sleep, they also lost their ability to regulate their body temperature. The longer they went without sleep the lower their temperature fell.

The inbuilt circadian rhythm also regulates body temperature. During the night, our body temperature falls one degree, whether we sleep or not. The temperature reaches its lowest point at the *nadir*, which is a kind of low point of the twenty-four-hour cycle – the opposite being the *zenith*. For most people, the nadir occurs two hours before we wake up, at around five in the morning. At that point, we are at our coldest – and sleepiest. It is as if our body, in consultation with the circadian rhythm, has decided that this is the point at which we have the greatest likelihood of being asleep – like when we set the thermostat on our house's heating system at the lowest temperatures for the times we are sure that everybody will be asleep or out for the day. Many people prefer to sleep in a cool room, and it has been demonstrated that this leads to better sleep. There is a natural explanation for this. The Earth's orbit around the sun doesn't just affect the light around us but also the temperature. Evolution has had to take into account not only the darkness, but also the cold of night. A bedroom where the atmospheric temperature is too high can disturb our nightly sleep.

People who work nights or who have decided to stay up when the rest of the world is asleep for other reasons will feel sleepiest at the nadir, and most traffic accidents that happen at night occur at around this time.

A hot bath before bedtime can help you sleep better. This isn't because the hot water makes you nice and warm; it is because of the *fall* in body temperature when the heat is extracted through the surface of your skin, streaming out as you step out of the bathtub. Your body grows colder – a signal that night has come.

Our body hurts when we don't get enough sleep. Muscles and joints ache, and wounds do not heal. Several important hormones that rebuild and fortify our body are produced during sleep. Cortisol is a hormone that affects our metabolism, enabling us to mobilise energy and better cope with physical strain. It is linked to stress but is also produced when we sleep. Production is at its lowest at bedtime, increases over the night and peaks when we wake up in the morning. Cortisol's production curve is opposite to that of melatonin.

During deep sleep, children and young people secrete growth hormones. Children with sleep problems who don't get enough deep sleep may stop growing. If they start to sleep deeply again later, growth can resume. But there are growth hormones for adults too. The skeleton is supplied with minerals, wounds are healed and other minor damage the body has suffered during the day is repaired. It has also been demonstrated that when cells are removed from the body – to be cultivated in a laboratory, say – division is most vigorous at night.

Appetite increases and alters with sleep deprivation; most people gain weight if they sleep too little for relatively long periods. The rat studies showed that sleep-deprived rats ate more than rats that were able to sleep and yet they lost body mass. This is linked to the unstable body temperature.

But appetite is also linked to processes in the brain. An American study monitored fourteen people over two four-day periods.[31] In the first period, they got a normal night's sleep and in the second, they got four hours' sleep. The researchers analysed the subjects' blood and hormone levels while also monitoring their eating habits. In the period of little sleep, the subjects experienced increased appetite, and several accepted the unhealthy supplementary food they were offered – even though they had eaten a meal a short time before. The study showed that sleep deprivation leads to an imbalance in both the hormone that signals satiety and the hormone that signals hunger. The feeling of satiety is muted, *and* the feeling of hunger is amplified. A sleep deficit also triggers the body's production of endocannabinoids, as happens when people smoke hash or marijuana, making them snack more. In addition, lack of sleep weakens the brain's impulse control, as demonstrated by an experiment conducted by Walker. He let the participants choose food based on pictures, first after a normal night and then after a wakeful night. During the experiments, the participants' brain activity was measured. The activity in what Walker calls the *supervisory regions* in the prefrontal cortex was silenced by a lack of sleep. The participants became more like children, lacking in impulse control, and allowed themselves to be guided by primal instincts rather than common sense and moderation.

A word to people who think it's macho to go to bed late and get up early: the libido diminishes and can disappear entirely if we don't get enough sleep. In one study, ten young men were made to sleep fewer than five hours a night over a fairly long period.[32] The fall in their testosterone level effectively 'aged' them by ten to fifteen years in terms of testosterone virility. And testosterone isn't just about libido; it also helps with energy levels and concentration. What's more, it contributes to greater bone density and muscle building. Sleeplessness places several obstacles in the way of those who wish to reproduce: a Danish study from 2013 showed that the sperm quality of men who slept little or poorly was 25 per cent lower than that of men who got enough sleep.[33] A Swedish study shows that too little sleep quite simply makes people less attractive. Healthy men and women aged between eighteen and thirty-one were photographed in a neutral setting, first after a normal night's sleep and then after thirty-one hours without sleep. When other people were asked to rank the photos by attractiveness, the images that were taken after the least amount of sleep consistently came out worst.[34] If this is true, it seems as though evolution is trying to get rid of the insomniacs, just as it has tried to weed out humans with other weaknesses: *Choose a different mate; this specimen can't even sleep.*

I can see and relate to the physiological changes caused by my own sleep deprivation. I can think: OK, but this is because I haven't had enough sleep. I can take precautions and wait until I am rested. It's worse when my brain starts to let me down, because then my capacity for judgement, oversight and rationality vanishes, to be replaced with confusion and desperation. Although I can suffer severe sleep deprivation several times a week, it feels as if I am drowning in my own life every single time. 'After sixteen hours of being awake, the brain begins to fail,' Walker writes. 'Humans need more than seven hours of sleep each night to maintain cognitive performance. After ten days of just seven hours of sleep, the brain is as dysfunctional as it would be after going without sleep for twenty-four hours. Three full nights of recovery sleep (i.e. more nights than a weekend) are insufficient to restore performance back to normal levels after a week of short sleeping. Finally, the human mind cannot accurately sense how sleep-deprived it is when sleep-deprived.'[35] Here Walker is talking about a brain with normal sleeping patterns. For me, seven hours of continuous sleep is something I can no longer imagine.

Studies have also shown that reduced sleep diminishes cognitive abilities; in other words our capacity to comprehend, think, learn, solve problems and remember. Without enough sleep, we perform more poorly on arithmetic problems, number recognition, speed, precision and short-term memory. In 2015, American researchers made one group of subjects go without sleep for sixty-two hours, while the other group slept normally. Both groups were asked to press a button when they were shown certain numbers. Then they were told to press the button when shown other numbers. Not one of the sleep-deprived subjects managed to do this without making a mistake – not even after forty attempts. Memory and sleep may form a vicious circle. There is a protein called beta-amyloid that scientists assume to be the cause of Alzheimer's disease. The more of this protein people have in parts of their brain, the less deep sleep they get. And the less deep sleep people get, the more difficult it is for them to get rid of this protein of forgetfulness

So, given how badly I sleep – are my chances of getting Alzheimer's higher?

Drifting through the day after too little sleep feels unbearable but is relatively harmless. It's worse if I sit behind the wheel of a car. Now and then, I'm able to grasp that I haven't had enough sleep to get behind a steering wheel; but often I'm in a grey zone. I've slept for a few hours and feel relatively rested – but enough to drive a car? Other times, I've driven when I should unquestionably have avoided it and, yes, with my children in the backseat. I don't think I would have fallen asleep at the wheel – as a rule that happens to drivers who have been awake for twenty-four hours or more and are suffering acute sleep deprivation. I drive to the kindergarten and to work, then home again; these are short trips without any long, monotonous stretches. If I have such great difficulty falling asleep at other times of day or night, why should it be so easy for me to drift off in the car? In these circumstances I'm much more likely to be affected by *micro-sleep*, which is something that happens to insomniacs who regularly get too little sleep. Micro-sleep is just what it sounds like: you sleep for a couple of seconds and then wake up again. Your eyes slide shut, the sensory doors are closed and for the blink of an eye – literally – you are blind and deaf and incapable of movement. Most people experience this in front of the TV just before bedtime. If you are sitting on an office chair or a sofa, micro-sleep can be an effective way of relaxing. But if you are sitting behind the wheel of a car, that little flicker of sleep is enough to place you and other people in grave danger. And even without micro-sleep, I shouldn't drive when I'm suffering from sleep deprivation. After fifteen to nineteen hours without sleep, our reaction time is diminished to the same extent as if we had a blood alcohol concentration of 0.08 per cent. Think of that next time you stay sober to drive other people home late at night.

IV

Since my insomnia arrived, I have allowed it to take on the starring role in my emotional life and have blamed it for my abrupt mood swings. But as I have grown older and the bad periods have become worse, I am no longer certain what is cause and what is symptom. Am I down because I'm not sleeping or, am I not sleeping because I am down?

Some years before I became chronically sleepless, I experienced insomnia for a short period, and on that occasion it was a symptom with an obvious cause. I was twenty-five and it was my last summer in Bergen. In May, I had taken my final exam in law. While I was looking for work and places on other courses, I worked as a waiter out at Verftet, on the Nordnes peninsula, which involved evening and night shifts. I met a girl and fell head-over-heels in love with her; after a matter of days I was ready to turn my life upside-down for her. Four weeks later, she left me for somebody else. I was twenty-five years old, but when it came to being in love I was still like a child, defenceless against my emotions and the confusion that raged inside me. All those night shifts had taken a toll on my circadian rhythm and I no longer knew whether it was early or late. And every night after work, I went out on the town and drank till I dropped. If I didn't drink, I'd lie awake thinking about where she was, who she was with. I would move from my bed to one sofa, then another sofa. (Ironically enough, in those days, I lived in a flat with five three-piece suites and six sofas.) I sweated, I froze. I'd put on one of the films from my tiny VHS collection, then another; it made me forget for a little while at least. When the film ended, the pain returned. And the thoughts. Everything that had been in my life before was still there. But because I had met this one person in the world, won her and then lost her, everything became worthless. A week went by, then two. I couldn't stop thinking about her, couldn't forget. Couldn't sleep. I was a beginner when it came to sleeplessness – didn't even understand that this *was* sleeplessness. I drank to sleep. The few bedtime routines I had – brushing my teeth, press-ups, reading a bit before I switched off the light – quickly vanished.

Only late into the morning, after the rush hour outside my living-room window ended, did I vanish into a light sleep, just for a few minutes or half an hour if I was lucky. Then I would shower, dress and walk through the city, across Nordnes and out to Verftet. I felt like an empty, see-through plastic bag plucked up by the wind, directionless and weightless.

The only thing anchoring me was my job out at Verftet. I opened the bar where I was on duty, prepared the till and the cigarettes and the coffee cups, the cutlery and the menus, and then I stood there waiting, drinking coffee to stay awake. Heartbreak and sleeplessness mingled, creating a physical pain in my chest that spread down into my belly and up into my throat.

A few weeks later I left Bergen. The depression lifted along with the sleeplessness.

In hindsight, this episode shows that I was already vulnerable when it came to sleep. If I became depressed, stressed or enthusiastic, my sleep was hardest hit.

One of my friends had a different experience in her student days, and for her it was the beginning of her sleep difficulties. When she started to study, she moved into a shared house with a friend, who soon succumbed to depression. My friend became so concerned and absorbed in her friend's crisis that *she too* fell into a crisis. Both dropped out after just half a year. She started to lie awake at night worrying about her friend. *There was one month when I didn't sleep,* she told me, *and in the end, I was the one with depression.* Her sleep difficulties and depression became so bad that she had to move back in with her parents. Eighteen years later she still struggles with insomnia.

Walker has studied sleep deprivation and the changes it causes in our emotional life. Brain scans of people who slept too little showed a 60 per cent increase in the activity of the amygdala – a part of the brain that plays an important role in triggering strong feelings such as anger.[36] Walker writes: 'It was as though, without sleep, our brain reverts to a primitive pattern of uncontrolled reactivity. We produce unmetered, inappropriate emotional reactions, and are unable to place events into a broader or considered context.' People who slept enough showed controlled, modest reactivity. Walker found that enough sleep led to a strong link between the amygdala, what he calls the *emotional gas pedal*, and the part of the brain that contributes to rational thought, the prefrontal cortex, the *brake*. When subjects slept too little, the link between these two regions was lost. There was too much gas and too little brake. When we sleep, we reinforce this link. If we sleep too little, we lose this delicate balance, as well as control over our emotions.

But sleep deprivation doesn't lead to exclusively negative emotions, either. Walker also noticed that the subjects could experience abrupt mood swings. They 'traversed enormous emotional distances,' as the sleep scientist puts it. One new study showed that another deep emotional centre, the striatum – which is linked to impulsivity and reward, and secretes the chemical dopamine – was hyperactive when the sleep-deprived person ended up in pleasurable situations, and that this hedonistic part of the brain, too, was going at full throttle, without any brake.[37] When we sleep too little, we risk being hurled to and fro between our own emotional extremes.

There is also an Italian study in which the researchers made people with bipolar disorder, who were in a stable period, spend a whole night awake. A large proportion of them immediately plunged into a manic period or a depressive episode.[38] This shores up Walker's assumption: that sleep deprivation is a trigger for, rather than a side effect of, mental disorders.

A Norwegian study shows that the link between sleep deprivation and depression goes both ways.[39] The study is based on roughly 25,000 participants who filled in two questionnaires at an interval of eleven years. They were asked about sleep difficulties, depression, physical ailments and other factors. The researchers found that the people who had insomnia at both points were six times more likely to be depressed at the end of the eleven years. At the same time, the people who had been depressed at both points were seven times more likely to have developed insomnia.

V

'That we are not much sicker and much madder than we are is due exclusively to that most blessed and blessing of all natural graces, sleep,' wrote Aldous Huxley. This is logical: we need rest to repair muscles, regulate our body temperature and maintain the body's capacity to withstand injury and disease. In the end, after more rats had suffered through further experiments, it turned out that what killed the sleep-deprived lab rats was not heat loss and lack of food but blood poisoning: a bacteria from the rats' bowels. An infection that a rested body would have dispatched quickly and easily.

But the fact that we must sleep to experience something as fundamental as a purposeful existence is the most merciless symptom and the greatest mystery of sleeplessness.

I clearly see the connection between psyche and sleep

in my children. With them, it alters from day to day, and the link between the sleep they've had and their behaviour the following day is obvious. If they go to bed early and sleep through the night they are, almost without exception, happy, confident and biddable. If they haven't had their dose of sleep, which is almost three times more than I need myself, I can already see the result in the first few minutes of the day. They may start to cry at the least opposition or react with tantrums where they would normally show tolerance and patience. But they can also switch directly from tears to laughter and then back to tears again. Most obviously, I see these strong emotions playing out in the two-year-old after a bad night. He has almost no control over his emotions to start off with, and without sleep he becomes helpless.

I know that these shifts within us are not controlled by sleep alone – a good day can follow a sleepless night and a bad day can follow a good night's sleep. Sometimes it feels as if sleep isn't at the wheel, but has been banished to the backseat, as if other forces are in control. In my bad periods, I start to doubt whether any of the things I'm doing in order to sleep better have any influence whatsoever on this rhythm. I exercise, I eat healthily, I cut out coffee and dim the bathroom light at night – and still I capsize. I cling onto the rudder but what good does that do when I'm caught up in currents beyond my control?

Night of Tuesday 21st June. Fall asleep in bed at 11.30 p.m., wake at 1 a.m. Go and lie on the sofa. Sleep around 3 a.m. Wake at 4 a.m. Last night's sleep: very light. Daytime functioning: very bad.

After six nights and days almost without sleep, it's as though the leaden cloak is lifted from me and the clenched fist in my midriff relaxes. Early in the afternoon I already have an inkling that the sleep I've been awaiting is finally on its way. Whether it's because the bad patch has reached its end or is down to sheer exhaustion – or both things combined – I don't know; but I recognise a shift in the balance that I will never understand but must always submit to.

Night of Wednesday 22nd June. I go to bed at 11 p.m., sleep at once and wake up at 6.30 a.m. Last night's sleep: very deep. Daytime functioning: very good.

This morning we take the bike, which has stood idle for the past week. I drop the children off at kindergarten and go to the Business School to write for an hour. It's been seven days since I last looked at my manuscript – I write one sentence, then another and then it's as if everything opens up and I vanish into the text. On my way to work on this summer morning, I breathe deep: my body is warm, my will strong. I am awake.

Before lunch, I ring Mum.

'I've been trying to get hold of you all week,' she says.

'I've had lots to do,' I say. 'But I've got some time now. Shall we sort out that trip?'

Then I send a mail to Andreas and apologise for not delivering the strips as agreed; I promise that twelve new ones will come during the evening and the rest tomorrow. I write the strips as I wait for my little girl to go to sleep. Line goes to bed early. It is still only 10 p.m.; I have the evening and the night ahead of me.

I open up my Mac and place my guitar on my lap.

JULY

The Journey

About how small children sleep and keep the rest of us awake; why teenagers have good reason to be tired in the morning; and the search for my own sleepless forebears.

I

Summer holidays. We have to catch an early flight out to Crete. I always sleep poorly the night before important early departures: lie down on the sofa at around midnight, doze off for a few hours but am up quarter of an hour before the alarm goes off. We wake the kids at three in the morning, get their clothes on and sit them in the car. Then we drive to the airport. It's night, dark and chilly – I see the disrupted sleep in their faces. But both of them realise we're on our way to something new and exciting, so they're keyed up and happy. On the plane, we all go to asleep, one after another; even I fall asleep, waking clear-headed after ten minutes.

We land at Chania airport around lunchtime and by early afternoon we're already in the hotel swimming pool. We're travelling with another family who have small children and although they are good friends who know about my sleep difficulties, Line and I have both been uneasy in the run-up to the trip because I've slept so badly in the past two weeks that we even considered cancelling. First of all because I've been on the brink of exhaustion from week after week without sleep; secondly because we have a certain responsibility for the other family's holiday too – I can't turn up in Crete like a zombie: it would cast a shadow over the whole party and that would be unbearable for both me and Line.

Hiding extreme sleep deprivation is something I'm good at, but always for a limited period – a working day, a night out with others. Pulling myself together all day every day when we're going to be spending two whole weeks in such close proximity – that's something I could never manage.

Despite all my efforts, my sleep difficulties haven't vanished; they have worsened. And it seems as though the good patches have changed too, becoming briefer, and my behaviour is much more manic. I can't get a grip on myself.

Before the holiday, I went to my GP to find out what had happened to the referral he'd sent. It was odd that I hadn't heard anything, he said, and sent another referral. I'm still hoping a sleep study will give me some answers.

I've packed my sleep books in my suitcase, the medical ones. I left the self-help books behind. I can't cope with any more advice and tips about putting down my mobile and exposing myself to daylight and going for walks.

Here we are in the southern Mediterranean and closer to the equator, where the sun sets more quickly – night falls in a matter of minutes. Since I've been up for eighteen hours and barely slept before then, I'm so sleepy the first evening that I barely manage to stay awake until the kids are in bed. Part of me is aware of all the risks: the pressure to 'perform' a good night's sleep so that the two families will have a pleasant day tomorrow; the new, unfamiliar hotel bed; the heat; the air-conditioning system – all these are factors that may keep me awake the whole night. Another part of me doesn't care. This night, fortunately, the indifferent side of me wins. That's the way sleep works: every night we have to forget all our worries, fears and joys, we have to set aside everything that livens up our existence in order to enter sleep. It doesn't matter whether we'll be leading a nation or robbing a bank the next day – sleep doesn't care. If we are to sleep, we must become passive, calm, biddable, submissive. Only then are we let in.

Next morning, I wake up at the same time as the children. I give them an iPad and a bowl of fruit then make myself a cup of instant coffee and sit out on the terrace.

The sense of being rested is like a caramel I savour throughout the day. I can feel the sleep working in me after the night – in my clear-headedness, body temperature, wellbeing, strength.

We eat breakfast together, the whole party, then pack our bags and walk the short distance down to the town beach, where we spend the morning. After that it's back to the hotel to eat lunch and carry on bathing in the pool. Whether it's the Mediterranean air, all the physical activity during the day, the freedom from stress and work; whether it's the early departure that's nudged my circadian rhythm back into place or whether it was simply time for a good patch – I don't know. But over the next days and weeks I sleep well, and those terrible days and nights before the departure are erased.

Only once the holiday is over and kindergarten and work resume in the last week of July do my problems return. The good patch has lasted so long I am taken by surprise.

O, sleeplessness!

Once more, I had hoped it was over. Once more the

disappointment and despair wash over me. To hope is also to open the door: anything can get in.

But my own sleeping difficulties aren't the only things that are back. It takes a long time to get the kids to bed on the first evenings after the holiday – they've become used to staying up late at night, and now it's nine or ten o'clock before they sleep. While Line settles the two-year-old, I try to chivvy the five-year-old through her nightly routines: supper, toothbrushing, toilet, reading, singing. The last thing I have to do before she closes her eyes is switch on the night-light. Although she has to be nagged the whole time, I know that every step in her nightly bedtime routines is important for her.

These routines are lost to me. While the children and Line have to go through a long series of tasks before they are ready for bed, as a rule I simply go and lie down. Some evenings, I don't even bother to get undressed. So obsessed am I with the bed and bedroom that everything must be in the right place. Yet the bedroom remains an ideal, an abstract. I never find my way in there.

For me, the borderline between day and night, bed and living room is erased. The lights in the living room may as well stay on all night. So what if I forget to brush my teeth? I won't get to sleep anyway.

The others prepare for sleep as if they were heading off on a long journey; I always leave open the possibility that I'll get no further than the front door or a little way down the road before having to turn back. I remember that I once had them, too, these rituals everybody goes through before settling for the night. As a child and some way into my teens I even offered up a little prayer to God before going to sleep, but it wasn't respect for the adults or God that made me carry on doing so: it was because I was meant to be going to sleep. No other rituals were so entrenched in me as those I carried out before night came. If I realised I had forgotten to go to the toilet before bedtime, I had to get up again – it didn't matter whether or not I actually needed to pee. Leaving out this one step in the evening routine, for even a single night, was impossible.

I see the same thing with my daughter. Although we have to remind her, from dawn to dusk, of all the things we want her to do, she always remembers her nightly routines. And if we grown-ups forget one of the steps, she stops us: aren't we going to read a story? She can't shut her eyes until everything is done. The routines are akin to obsessive thoughts, but they help her and everybody else to sleep.

Soon both children are asleep but the night has barely begun. When at last I feel sleep approaching at around one o'clock, the two-year-old wakes up, just as I am dozing off. I curse, hurry to him and try to get him back to sleep, but fail to hide my own desperation because I know that now I'll have to wait at least another hour, maybe more, before getting another try – if indeed a fresh chance comes at all. I must hide my frustration. The boy, half asleep, half awake, must be soothed if he is to get back to sleep; he'll notice if I'm angry or stressed and that will only rouse him further and then it will take more time to get him back to sleep. I stand over his bed and stroke his neck until he quietens. Soon I hear his heavy breathing. He is sleeping deeply.

I go into our bedroom and put my duvet under my arm. Line wakes up and looks at me.

'Where are you going?'

'The kids woke me up. I'm going to lie on the sofa.'

I go up to the TV room, put on a film – something that will engage me just enough so I can follow it, but won't engage me too much – and lie down. At two o'clock I'm woken up from a deep sleep: this time it's the five-year-old who's had one of her night-time episodes. I hurry down to her before she can wake the others, but it's too late. Her screams have also woken Line. The only thing we know of that helps is to give her an iPad and let her watch a film until she calms down. Half an hour later, we can switch off the film and tell her to shut her eyes. She falls asleep. It's 2.40 a.m. Unbelievably enough I manage to fall asleep again on the sofa before being woken up once more by one of the children whimpering loudly. I look at my watch, 4.30 a.m., put on a new film, then sleep lightly until six o'clock when the boy wakes and wants to get up. He's tired and whiny, has slept too little; even though I lie down beside him in his bed, I can't get him back to sleep again. He frets and wants to get up because he isn't old enough to grasp that he's sad because he hasn't had enough sleep. So, it's up and on with the day, with all that this implies.

II

If my own sleep difficulties are the Western Front, the children are the Eastern Front. The territory I am trying to defend, my own sleep, is becoming ever smaller. The first thing I worried about when I found out we were going to have our first child was how sleeping would go. My own, of course, not Line's or the child's. A newborn in the house, screaming by night and sleeping by day: that would further complicate my efforts to get any sleep. What I really feared was all the changes a child would bring. By then, I had been struggling with sleep for ten years. I didn't sleep, feared both night and day, and felt

I never had enough control to shut my eyes and relax. For me, the quest for sleep has always been intimately linked to the quest for predictability. The insomniac is waiting for catastrophe to strike. The moments in life when I lose my footing are always the times when I also lose sleep. New job, new places, concerts, book launches – that's when I always lie awake. Only when everything in life has fallen into place have I been able to sleep. And every time I've been heading towards something new, I've always thought: *This won't work. I'm not even sleeping at night; I have enough to do just coping with myself – I can't deal with this too.* (Convincing oneself that everything affects one's own sleep is, after all, the principal task of the insomniac.)

As Line's belly grew, the attention we had devoted to me and my sleep difficulties diminished. Line had enough on her hands just getting to work and back. Her thoughts were on the birth and the early days with the child. She didn't have time to nurse my neuroses; she didn't have time to help me find peace at night or to ask me about my sleep in the mornings. What she needed now was a man who was present and – sleep or no sleep – *functional*.

Negative emotions, whether minor worries or deep anxieties, depend on attention. Now nobody had any time for my sleep-related anxieties – not even me – it was as if the vicious circle was broken. At first I slept just as poorly as before, but when morning came I shrugged it off and started my day. I had a heavily pregnant wife; who had time to hear about sleep disorders?

When our daughter came into the world, I was outside myself for the first time in my adult life. It was no longer all about me: now I was there for other people. The cycle my thoughts had followed for so long – my needs, my fears – ceased. My fear of not sleeping no longer merited attention.

We came home with our first child, gave her food and laid her down to sleep in a crib we had set up in the living room. I crept around the house to avoid waking mother and child. Everything now revolved around the fundamental needs: food and sleep. But not my food – and not my sleep. During these early weeks and months with a newborn in the house, I slept better than I had for many years. The cat padding around me in circles – I didn't give a damn whether it settled in my lap or not. I had more important things on my mind. The dove beside my hand – it could fly away or stay, I didn't have time for it now. My self-consciousness, hitherto in control, vanished almost entirely. The ironic process of mental control was halted, the vicious circle was broken. I slept.

III

I sleep like a baby, I'm up every two hours, says insomniac American comic Billy Crystal. We use children as a symbol of long, undisturbed sleep, but the fact is that it's quite the opposite: newborns are like wild horses when it comes to sleep – they must be tamed and trained in the established sleeping pattern of the society into which they are born. Nothing is more disruptive to the sleeping patterns of adults than having a newborn in the house.

And yet the proportion of REM sleep is at its highest during the last weeks before we are born; we never reach those levels again.[40] In adolescence, we get more deep sleep than at any time later in life, but then it starts to abate. At around thirty, a significantly smaller part of the night is spent in deep sleep. And the deep sleep we do get is not as deep as before, either. Before we have made it through our forties, we have lost 60–70 per cent of the deep sleep we had in our adolescence, and by the time we turn seventy, we have lost 80–90 per cent. This doesn't imply that we *need* less sleep; it simply means that it is more difficult for us to get it.

As newborns, we have no circadian rhythm. Only towards the end of the first year of our life is our biological clock fully developed, allowing us to track the passage of the light and the day. By the age of four, we are capable of staying up all day and sleeping all night. But our circadian rhythm will be disrupted several times before we reach adulthood. The child is ahead of the adult in its circadian rhythm – children both sleep and wake earlier. This changes for teenagers: their circadian rhythm lags some hours behind the normal one. Young people who stay awake at night and struggle to get up in the morning are actually at the mercy of their genes. Walker has proposed the theory that this lagging circadian rhythm is a tool whose purpose is to help teenagers break away from adults by giving them a couple of hours in their own company and that of other adolescents.[41]

If he develops normally my two-year-old son will sleep more continuously the older he becomes. Today, he wants to get up at six o'clock. In ten or eleven years, we won't be able to get him up in the morning – he'll do what all other teenagers do: sit up at night and sleep away the day. Then he will be incorporated into adult society and must work. His circadian rhythm will be shifted again, this time backwards, making it easier to get up in the morning, and he'll become sleepy earlier at night. And later in life, if he has a family, he will have to alter this circadian rhythm too, getting up at five o'clock to watch Peppa Pig with his own children. As he grows older, he will then get less and less deep sleep. He will follow the sleeping patterns all normal humans go through in life.

I hope.

The fact that I sleep badly increases the risk that my children will sleep badly. Insomnia can be hereditary, with an estimated transmission rate of 28–45 per cent from parent to child.[42] In that case, sleeplessness is hidden deep within them – maybe it won't strike until they reach adulthood, as it did for me. Even now I'm on the lookout for signs: whether they fall asleep quickly or take a long time to do so; whether they sleep heavily or lightly. How much do they sleep over the day and night? Is it normal?

To answer these questions, I also have to look backwards. If what I suffer from is hereditary, who did I inherit it from?

IV

Sleep wasn't something that was talked about when I was a child, perhaps simply because there was enough of it. I was surrounded by adults who slept, and I quickly learnt to respect sleepers. I remember the afternoon naps at home with my grandparents on Dad's side. After dinner, they would lie down, each on their own sofa, each in their own room: Grandma on the green plush sofa in the parlour and Grandpa in the living room with the open fire. And then there must be silence. I was given cushions and a blanket on the floor, midway between the two rooms, and there I lay, listening to their snoring and the tick of the clock out in the hall. Sometimes I slept too, just for a moment, but it was enough to get that feeling of a scene change a brief nap can give us.

Then the house woke up again to the TV news, while Grandma switched on the rest of the lights, brewed the coffee and brought out little cakes. Grandma was a chatty, lively woman who cherished those around her. She had a carefree manner and, although I didn't think about this during childhood, I am convinced she was a person who slept well at night, like her son, my father. Nobody sleeps better and longer than Dad. He can lie in till late in the morning, take an hour's afternoon nap and settle for the night early in the evening.

Grandpa, the grandparent I spent most time with, tended to worry more. He didn't seem to take anything lightly: he thought about everything and everyone. When I was in hospital having the stitches taken out after an appendectomy, he stood beside my bed and wept with me. Sometimes when I spent the night at theirs, he would sleep in the lower bunk and we would lie there chatting together until I fell asleep.

'Are you hungry?' he would ask.

'No,' I'd say.

'Good. It isn't easy to sleep on an empty stomach.'

He gave me an alarm clock because I'd need it to get up in the morning. It was a huge, old-fashioned model in bronze-coloured metal, with two bells on top and a hammer in between that woke the entire house when it started to vibrate. It ticked loudly, too loudly, and many nights I had to put it in the wardrobe muffled with clothes if I wanted to sleep, otherwise I'd lie there listening to the ticking. It seemed to increase in intensity as I waited for it to go off.

I don't know whether or not Grandpa slept well at night – I never asked him. When you're a child, sleep is something you move in and out of, with ease and without giving it any thought.

My maternal grandfather took his after-dinner nap in a chair in a corner, newspaper on his lap – just sat there snoring. Grandmother was a thin, transparent woman and undoubtedly the most nervous of my four grandparents. Did she sleep well at night? My two uncles were both bachelors in their twenties when I was a little boy and on Saturdays and Sundays they would sleep until late in the afternoon. Sometimes, we might come to dinner to find Grandmother boiling potatoes while Uncle Øyvind lay up in the loft, still fast asleep. He ate dinner in his pyjamas!

And then there were all the different places I spent my nights as a child. There was the bunk bed at home, where I slept on top and my brother down below. Later, I got my own room, where I slept on a zebra-striped sofa bed. On the mornings when I could be bothered, I'd pull open a big drawer, stuffing in the duvet, pillow and sheet before shutting the drawer again and arranging the three zebra-patterned cushions on top of the sofa. At Grandma and Grandpa's house I would also sleep in the upper bunk bed, where Dad and his brother had slept as children. Over the bed hung a poster of the Tower of London with drawings of Beefeaters, which I might lie and study before falling asleep and just after waking. At Grandmother and Grandfather's house, I spent the early years sleeping on a mattress at the foot of their double bed and later slept in a box bed in the loft in Uncle Øyvind's boyhood room, with posters of Pink Floyd, Genesis and Deep Purple on the walls. When we went on road trips down through Europe, Dad would convert the back seat into a big bed with garden cushions and blankets. This was obviously before parents started worrying about child safety in cars, because here my brother and I lay and slept our way through Northern

Europe. Now and then we'd stop off en route to visit friends of my parents. We would arrive late at night and then we semi-slumbering boys would be carried out of the car and laid down on an unfamiliar mattress in an unfamiliar living room. I used to go on camping trips to Hamar and Sweden with Grandma and Grandpa, and then I would spend the night in a bunk bed in their camper van, mere centimetres between my nose and the roof. Before going to sleep, I would lie up there looking down at what was happening in the cramped camper van: at Grandma and Grandpa sitting watching Swedish news and boxing matches. In the morning, I'd wake up drenched in sweat; the tiny space where I'd spent the night became hot as a roasting oven the minute the sun struck the roof. In summer, we'd sometimes pitch a tent in the back garden, too, and there we'd be allowed to spend the night, my brother and I, later with pals. We took out groundsheets, sleeping bags, crisps, drinks, torches and comics. Then we lay awake until late into the night. These sleepovers with friends are my first memories of not getting to sleep. I was always the last one to settle and even then I'd lie awake, nose to the damp tent canvas, listening to the insects outside and the deep breathing from the sleeping bags around me.

After my parents divorced, I got two rooms and two beds. At first my brother and I slept in a bunk bed in the same room as Dad, then we each got our own room in a bigger flat. In the end, I moved into Dad's new house on a mountainside overlooking Ellingsøy Fjord. I had a big attic room with a dormer window where I slept on a blue sofa bed, and during the autumn storms the rain would lash my window as the wind snatched at the wall beside my bed.

During childhood, I had several lengthy hospital stays,

first with appendicitis, later with volvulus – a twisted loop of intestine. On the last occasion I was placed in quarantine, which involved lying alone in a bare room while all my visitors had to wear suits, hoods and masks. When night fell, I had to be alone. Mum would spend the evenings with me but then she, too, had to leave. I'd stand by the window weeping as I looked at her down there in the car park. And I can still remember the feeling of being woken early in the morning by a nurse, then having to get out of bed and sit in a chair, so tired I could barely hold my eyes open, as I waited for my bedclothes to be changed.

My class went on a camping trip, fifteen lads in the same dormitory, and although I wasn't the worst of them, I was always among the culprits when the teacher had to come in during the night to deal with the noise. The more tired I got, the wilder I became. In the company of other boys, I'd do whatever it took to fit in and this lack of social self-reliance seemed to manifest itself most clearly when I slept over with other boys, maybe because everything became so amplified when we were left to ourselves as children, lying close beside each other in the darkness. My greatest fear was exclusion. So if somebody got out of bed to make mischief, I'd join in or encourage them. When it came to keeping a bad joke going the entire night – generally at the expense of one of my classmates – I was in.

At thirteen, I began drinking: whatever me and my pals could sneak from our parents to start off with; then, later, the beer we'd get older boys to buy for us at the off licence. I drank everything and I drank a lot. In my early adolescence, I might knock back twelve beers in a matter of hours. The aim was total oblivion. Now and then I'd keep it going until the next day; grey-blue pre-dawn hours down at the seashore before the sun came up behind the mountains, sitting drunk and happy on a bare rock. The next day, I wouldn't get dressed until dusk fell outside, then I'd go down to the kitchen and have a bite to eat before crawling back up to my room and lying down, slipping in and out of sleep until night came and I could sleep no more.

At eighteen I did my military service. All that year, I slept in a six-man room, lying in one of the upper bunks the way I'd got used to in childhood. Five other eighteen-year-old lads chatting, laughing, snoring and groaning – it'd be a nightmare for me today. The days started at six o'clock and were filled with physical activity. If I sat still for five minutes I became drowsy. I'd lie down to sleep whenever I could, like a good soldier; it didn't matter when or where. The room could be full of noisy recruits knocking back soft drinks, I'd sleep through it all, pressing myself into the wall and making myself invisible so the others wouldn't wake me.

During the eight years I spent as a student – six in Bergen and two in Volda – I stepped out of society and also, as a result, out of a regular daily routine. It was like being hurled into a vacuum, without duties. Curriculum, assessments and marks were concepts I related to only in the final weeks before any exam; the rest of the time, I lived out a freedom so total that it ended up hamstringing me. I could lie in until two o'clock in the afternoon on Monday, go to a party on Tuesday and practise with my band all night on Wednesday. I'd often lie in my bed thoroughly keyed up, not wanting to sleep, just to carry on. But when sleep arrived at last, I slept deep and long.

In childhood, life is an endless series of changes, new endings and new beginnings. A new class, a new school, a new leisure activity, a new summer job, a holiday. Then maybe there's military service, studies and new jobs, new people to meet. This concentrated upheaval I experienced early in life is something I could never tackle now. I've become too old, too sensitive, too strongly attached to predictability. Those nights before something new, almost always Sunday nights, I would lie awake the whole night, irrespective of whether I was dreading getting up at six o'clock to go to a new warehouse job I'd rather get out of, or looking forward to going on holiday, or had an exam the next day – I was awake regardless and in the morning I would get up, hot and muddle-headed, with a fizzing sensation in my body. But it never struck me that lying awake throughout the night was a disorder or a disease. That came later.

Was it only when I gave sleeplessness a name and a place in my life that it began to cast its shadow? Did the disease arrive with the diagnosis? This was one of the reasons I was afraid to go to the doctor at first – I feared that by giving attention to my sleep difficulties I might feed them, make them grow. This is the self-obsessed human's curse: the more I prod at it, the more it hurts.

My brain is like a wilful child who refuses to obey. And what are we supposed to do with wilful children? A responsible adult carries on as before, ensuring that the child adjusts their behaviour. What have I done? I have stopped dead and tried to understand the wilful child – analysed, studied, *written* about the child. Maybe in my efforts to get better I have made everything worse.

The second week after the holiday, the nights are calmer. The boy still wakes at around one o'clock each night and although he wakes us every time, he quickly settles again.

94

I lie there on tenterhooks, waiting for all hell to break loose. Then one night, three weeks after the holiday, we sleep well and long, all four of us, not waking until 7.30 a.m. Everybody is calm, harmonious. I feel so rested that I'm not even bothered by the letter that finally arrives in the post. After more than three months, the response to my GP's referral has come. 'Based on the information we have received,' it reads, 'we have concluded that you are not entitled to the examination or treatment in the specialist health service. Grounds: No service available.'

AUGUST

All the Others

About acupuncture, criteria for insomnia and how sleep fell out of favour in the Enlightenment, giving us the armchair.

I

The underground carriage is full of Chinese tourists with selfie-sticks. I catch myself wondering if they're jetlagged or whether they sleep soundly in their hotel rooms somewhere in the city. As I go out into the dark, chilly subterranean corridors, I sweat; as I climb up to street level and the blazing sun, I start to freeze. The bustle of the city streets feels like an assault: the racket of street musicians, the chat of passers-by, the beeping of a truck as it reverses through the crowd on Øvre Slottsgate, the sunlight piercing my eyes, the late summer smell of mozzarella cheese and city dust. It's on days like this that I understand how much my brain allows me to ignore when I've had enough sleep; only a fraction of what happens around me attracts my attention. Of the rest, my brain seems to say: I won't trouble you with this. It isn't like that today. In the traffic, surrounded by so many people and moving vehicles, my sleepless brain fails me. It's incapable of sorting all the information coming from all directions and everything seems equally hazardous. I walk about in a constant state of preparedness, my personal space expands, and I am at war with anybody who comes within a five-metre radius. If I were walking here with the kids, it would be a nightmare trying to keep them in check.

I go past Spikersuppa and down towards the square outside City Hall, stopping on Roald Amundsens gate to look around. What was the address? I take out my mobile and check the note with the address on. Fridtjof Nansens plass. Placing two streets named after Norwegian polar explorers in such close proximity is bound to confuse insomniacs with diminished cognitive abilities. I type the address into the map app on my mobile but forget the numbers and have to try again. When I'm short of sleep, I'm forgetful to the point of danger. I lose my trolley at the supermarket, forget all the items I left on the car roof, can't be trusted to use drain cleaner alone: I'll pour it down the drain and end up leaving it there overnight.

The blue dot lights up on the map – it's really close by. I lift my gaze and place one foot in front of the other. I find the entrance in the shadow of City Hall, ring on the doorbell and press my ear against it to be sure I'll catch the sound of the lock. Some seconds later it buzzes and I lean against the door and push it open.

The waiting room and the rest of the premises are old and tatty, a far cry from the mellow, bright, clean web pages that appeared when I googled sleep difficulties and acupuncture. *Get results based on scientific knowledge and clinical experience*, ran the advert for this place, which offers chiropractic treatment, massage, physiotherapy, osteopathy and acupuncture. It's the last of these I'm here for. I know almost nothing about acupuncture other than it involves sticking needles into your body. I'm scared of needles – it seems so radical yet so arbitrary: like, *we'll stick one in here* – and I'm afraid one of the needles could hit a nerve or some other vital part. As long as they don't stick one in my forehead.

My name is called out and a woman in surgical green stands in the doorway of the waiting room. I get up and we greet each other. Her name is Gry and she leads me into a room with a couch in the centre and a desk by the window. In one corner there is a chair. I sit down.

First a chat, then needles.

'Would you say you are warm-blooded or cold-blooded?' Gry asks.

'When I haven't slept, I freeze and sweat by turns. If I've slept well, I warm up easily.'

'Do you drink coffee?'

'I drink a lot of coffee, but none after lunch.'

'Do you exercise?'

'I try, but I find it hard to get into a regular routine. Mostly because of my sleep difficulties.'

'How would you describe yourself?'

Giving an account of oneself to strangers is like drawing lots: a new person with new qualities emerges every time. I give it some thought. 'A bit intense, maybe. Social. Talkative, sometimes.'

'Do you brood?'

'Not really. Or rather, yes. But not when I'm trying to get to sleep at any rate.'

The acupuncturist nods and smiles. She often laughs when I answer; seems to be bubbling over. She's easy to talk to, with a dialect from some place north of my hometown, Nordmøre or Romsdal.

'This is what I specialised in when I was studying,' she says. 'So I find it very interesting.'

'You specialised in sleep difficulties? At acupuncture school?'

I don't know if this is the correct description of her training, but she nods.

'There's one centre in the body for fight or flight, and another for the opposite. I'll focus on these two and try to move them further apart. That way, we'll re-establish the balance in your body.'

She gets up.

'Now you can take off your shoes and socks and lie on the couch.'

I make myself comfortable. She lifts up my left arm and takes my pulse, then asks to see my tongue, which I stick out reluctantly. Is she going to stick the first needle in there? She leans over me and grips my tongue between two fingers. Then releases it.

'Fine. I just wanted to take a peek. Sometimes very anxious people get red dots on their tongues. Let's start with the needles.'

My whole body tenses in anticipation of the first needle. It'll probably hurt even more with tense muscles, I think. Gry stands behind me, by my head, leaning over me. She places a needle straight in my forehead. A brief white heat and then it's sitting there. She places one in my scalp and then continues down my body. One in each hand, in the flesh between thumb and index finger, and three in each foot.

'Can you feel that?' she asks. 'It's normal for it to hurt more the further away from the centre of the body you get.'

'The one in my forehead is worst.'

'Interesting.'

When all the needles are in and I'm lying there, she asks whether I want a blanket over me. I decline; I'm cold but I'm also afraid that the blanket will weigh on the needles and push them further into my body. Gry asks if I want some music and I say yes. She says it's nice to have something to focus on and puts on some music it is absolutely impossible to focus on. Then she leaves the room and I lie there alone staring at the ventilation system in the ceiling. The music is low so I can hear everything going on around me: a conversation between two men on the other side of the wall; a telephone ringing; the roar of traffic outside. For the first few minutes I just lie there, feeling the needles; I lift my right arm cautiously to look at the foreign body protruding from my flesh. What are these needles supposed to be good for? The only thing I know is that it's an ancient Chinese treatment that involves sticking needles into certain parts of the body to cure disease and promote health. Whether it works or is simply nonsense is a matter of controversy, as I realised when I read the Norwegian Wikipedia entry about acupuncture: even *the article itself* is controversial, the website administrator notes. But acupuncture holds out the prospect of a treatment for sleep difficulties – so here I am. Just bear with it, I think; in half an hour the needles will be out of your body and your body will be out of the building. And I don't have to come back.

Gry comes in again.

'Have you found peace?'

'Yes, I'm starting to notice it now.'

I always feel obliged to give strangers the answer they want, but this time it's true. The peace is coming.

'It's strange how calm you can feel with all those needles in your body,' Gry laughs, before leaving again.

No way on earth am I going to sleep now, I think as I feel myself growing drowsy. It's exactly like Daniel Wegner's experiment with marching music. If I *should* sleep, I'm not very likely to manage it. If I *must* sleep, it's impossible. But the pressure can be reversed. Once more, my brain reacts like a rebellious four-year-old: *You're not allowed to sleep, you hear?* Like now, in an unfamiliar office near City Hall with ten needles stuck in my body and an Enya tune that never seems to get going.

Bjorvatn writes about a patient with insomnia, a young student who lies awake for several hours every night before dozing off.[43] He attributes his sleep problems to his parents' divorce when he was thirteen; he used to lie awake listening to arguments and noise, and never managed to sleep before the house fell quiet. When the doctor asks him whether he can remember the last time he had a good night's sleep, he talks about a climbing trip he took with friends. Darkness fell before they reached the top and they were forced to attach themselves to the cliff for the night. Midway up the rock face, suspended in an uncomfortable position, he slept better than he had for ages.

I wake up when the door opens. The acupuncturist picks up my left hand and checks it. I come to; it's like climbing up to the surface, to oxygen and sunlight. I wake up out of sleep, but at the same time I emerge from my sleeplessness. My body is warm and doesn't hurt, my head is clear. A few minutes' sleep was all I needed.

'Did you sleep?'

'I think so.'

Why don't I just say yes? Is my need to make sleep more complicated than it is part of the problem? Or is it that I'm scared to admit that the acupuncture treatment has had the effect I was wishing for?

I get dressed. The acupuncturist sits at the PC again. She says she'll send me an e-mail with some tips about diet; food that will help me sleep better.

'Then I'll set up a new appointment for you next Tuesday. It's important to continue the treatment to get the full effect. It would be best to come a couple of times a week from now on.'

She looks at me and smiles.

'OK,' I say.

Two days later, I'm frying sausages and mashing potatoes for dinner when I get an e-mail from Gry. 'Tips and advice', it says in the subject line. 'Foods that are suitable for you and your problem: cucumber, broccoli, peas, cabbage, celery (especially for sleep), seafood (especially shellfish and octopus/squid), mutton, fennel, sesame seeds, sunflower seeds, wheat, saffron, thyme, grapes and water melon.'

I look down at the food I'm preparing, the glistening sausages writhing in the pan, the yellowish-white mashed potato, streaked golden from the butter I'm mixing in. On the table, I've already set out ketchup and mustard. Not the world's healthiest meal but one that all the family will eat until they are full.

Should I cut out sausages? I think. Eat squid, octopus and celery from now on? What about the rest of the family? Will they get the same?

How far should I go?

After dinner, I cancel the next acupuncture session. Instead I message a friend. *How's it going with the sleeping?*

The answer comes back fast: *Better.*

II

Njål is the only other sleepless person I know. We lived and studied together at a time some years before my own sleep difficulties burst into full bloom. There was drinking and partying until late almost every night – a time and a place where it wasn't easy to distinguish between people who didn't *want* to sleep and those who weren't *able* to sleep. The first I heard of Njål's problems was when his parents came to take him home one day. He was sleeping so badly at night that he had to take a sleeping cure, and that was impossible to do in a party pad in Volda. It struck me as much more serious than it really was. Njål might as well have been shipped off to the mental hospital – what was *really* wrong with him, I wondered? Two years later, I started lying awake at night myself.

I ask if he wants to meet up and talk about our sleep difficulties over a beer. We know about each other's insomnia but have never talked about it all that much, and never one on one. We are Western Norwegian men: it doesn't come naturally to us to sit exchanging anecdotes about illnesses. But now I want to know more. How did it start with Njål? How is it today? What has he done to improve matters? And that sleeping cure sixteen years ago – what was it? Is it something I ought to try?

Njål asks if we can have a beer on Friday or Saturday. Alcohol keeps him awake and he needs a day off to recover. At last, I thought, I can arrange a meeting based on the premise of insomnia, because that's exactly how it is for me too. I can manage one beer, but if I drink more than that I may lie awake the entire night. There's a reason why most alcoholics suffer from insomnia. At first alcohol has a tranquilising effect, which can help us fall asleep. But when the alcohol is on its way out of the bloodstream again, it has the opposite effect. Our pulse rate increases, we get less REM sleep than normal, our sleep becomes more superficial and is interrupted more frequently. If we do manage to sleep, the alcohol can cause violent dreams and nightmares in the latter part of the night. As if that weren't enough, alcohol relaxes the muscular activity in our pharynx, which leads to snoring and sleep apnoea and even more broken sleep. My solution is either to drink so much that I anaesthetise myself and postpone the withdrawal for many hours; then I sleep and don't wake until dawn. The alternative is to simply accept that I am heading for a sleepless night, since that is the price I must pay for having a social life. So many times I have sat there with a friend who decides to have that second beer, which I know will ruin my night, and all too often, I choose the beer over the night's sleep. For me, it's not about the alcohol but about trying to live normally.

As I sit waiting for Njål on Friday afternoon, I get a message: *Running late. Slept in.* Insomniac humour. Then he comes in, buys himself a beer and sits down. We start by exchanging rules: neither of us drinks coffee after a certain time in the afternoon. We both avoid certain kinds of screen use in the later hours, things that wind us up. Njål can't watch comedies; I can't watch horror movies. He has to sleep with earplugs. And he can't sleep with another person in his bed. He's in the process of breaking this last rule; Njål has found himself a new girlfriend and for the first time it looks as if sharing a bed with somebody is working fine.

While my life has a clear division between before and after insomnia, Njål has *always* been troubled by sleeplessness. It started long before he moved to Volda. He began to notice it himself when he was at secondary school, although according to his mother he'd had sleep problems at primary school too. In sixth form it gradually got worse, yet nothing was done about the problems.

'I'm a doctor's son,' Njål says. 'And that means you're never ill. It wasn't until I got to Volda that I started to deal with it.'

'But what sparked it, do you think?'

Njål shrugs.

'When I was supposed to be doing basic military service, I had to see a psychologist to get an exemption because of my sleep problems. She wanted an explanation too. If I was sleeping badly, there had to be some underlying issue, that was kind of the way of thinking. *Are you having a tough time? Don't you have any friends? What's wrong?* But I had nothing to show; I had a great childhood. There wasn't any trauma there.'

'I'm looking for the big reason, too,' I say.

Njål ponders.

'So, it must be the radio.'

'The radio?'

'I'd lie in bed listening to radio shows. I'd never lie there under the duvet thinking *now I'll relax*. It was a time for fantasising and thinking and pondering.'

Njål tells me he recently spent three weeks in New York, where he slept really badly. His gaze flickers slightly, his fingers wander up to his face as he speaks. We have the same nervous energy. Two emotional, ambitious, sleepless Western Norwegians who don't like to talk about emotions, ambitions or sleeplessness.

'Did you know we have an inbuilt circadian rhythm that makes it easier to travel west than east?' I ask.

I've read so much about sleep and sleep disorders lately that I can't drop the subject. But Njål doesn't rise to the bait.

'It wasn't because of jetlag,' he says. 'I was staying at a hotel. I'm always totally fucked at hotels.'

'Same here.'

'But on the plane I slept fine.'

'I always do too – like a baby. Planes, trains, buses. All the places where I'm not supposed to sleep,' I say.

'Maybe it's a kind of Pavlovian reaction to the bed,' Njål says.

'Pavlov's dogs started drooling at the sound of bells,' I say. 'We hear bells and manage *not to drool*.'

I ask him about that time in Volda when he went home to sort out his sleep difficulties; what did he do then?

'Dad knew a therapist who could treat me. He put me on a sleeping cure.'

'But what did it involve?'

'Sleep restrictions,' Njål says. 'Which means you're not allowed to sleep.'

'You're not allowed to sleep?'

'Well, you're allowed to sleep, but only a limited number of hours every night. And I had to sit in front of lamps, too.'

'Did it help?'

'A bit.'

Talking with another insomniac makes it easier to see my sleeplessness from the outside. A large part of not sleeping is self-deception because everything is so intangible, but now it feels as if the fog is lifting. For example, when Njål complains about how poorly he slept in New York, I suddenly remember the time I went there with my band to play some gigs and we lived in the city centre for eight weeks and I *didn't sleep*. This was many years before I developed chronic insomnia. Both before and after this trip, I slept well no matter where I was, but Manhattan was too much for me. I remember lying in an upper bunk at the YMCA on Seventh Avenue and staring at the ceiling, night after night after night.

Later in the evening, we are joined by Jørgen, a mutual acquaintance.

'Sleeplessness,' he sighs when he hears what we're talking about. 'It's a fad.'

Njål and I stop dead and look at him.

'What do you mean?'

'It's turned into a thing. It's like everybody's supposedly sleeping so badly,' Jørgen continues, and starts to rattle off people he knows who, according to him, *claim* to sleep badly. Njål and I burst out laughing and ask Jørgen how *he* sleeps.

'Ten hours every night, twelve to thirteen at the weekends,' he answers. 'And I usually have an hour's nap in the afternoon, too.'

I take out my notebook and pen.

'Those names,' I say. 'Can you repeat them?'

III

Marilyn Monroe suffered from insomnia and took sleeping pills. Napoleon became sleepless when stressed, which I assume happens frequently if you're trying to conquer Europe. Michael Jackson also suffered from insomnia. Propofol, the substance he eventually had too much of and died from, was what he used to sleep. Abraham Lincoln went for long nocturnal walks to combat his sleeplessness; Cary Grant had sleep difficulties and got up in the middle of the night to read. Benjamin Franklin shifted between two beds in his efforts to get some sleep. Theodore Roosevelt drank cognac and milk to overcome his insomnia. The actress Tallulah Bankhead paid other people to hold her hand so that she could get to sleep. If Marcel Proust hadn't had insomnia, he might never have written books. Vincent van Gogh was so desperate that he poured turpentine over his mattress. *Sleep is for wimps,* was the motto of the sleepless Margaret Thatcher. Charles Dickens wandered the streets of London at night. Sir Isaac Newton slept poorly, while Thomas A. Edison kept a sleep journal because of his sleep difficulties. Mark Twain, Franz Kafka, Alexandre Dumas, Vladimir Nabokov – all of them were sleepless, as are Patti Smith, Joni Mitchell and Madonna. Even Jimi Hendrix struggled with insomnia. The American author Chuck Palahniuk often fantasises about challenging somebody to a fistfight – and losing – in order to sleep. The comedian Groucho Marx suffered from insomnia: what do you get if you cross an insomniac, an agnostic and a dyslexic? *Someone who stays up all night wondering if there is a Dog.*

Between 2001 and 2011, the percentage of adult Norwegians with insomnia rose from 12 to 15.5 per cent.[44] Based on the National Statistics Office's population figures, that means more than 413,000 Norwegians had insomnia at the turn of the millennium. Ten years later, the figure had risen to almost 590,000. How many there are today we do not know, but there are good reasons to believe that the total is even higher.

Insomnia can affect anybody – not just celebrities. On the contrary, sleep problems are more common in the lower socioeconomic strata of the population. Reliable, conscientious, ambitious people who are easily worried are more prone to insomnia than others. We can also shelve the myth that people with good consciences sleep soundly: it's people *without* a conscience who sleep best. People who are well intentioned, with an exaggerated capacity for sympathy, those who are responsible and easily worried are more prone to insomnia, says sleep scientist Bjørn Bjorvatn. Walker writes: 'The two most common triggers of chronic insomnia are psychological: 1) emotional concerns, or worry, and 2) emotional distress, or anxiety.'[45]

Between 2 and 30 per cent of all children aged six months to two years suffer from sleeplessness (according to the children's parents, who are the only people in a position to diagnose them, after all). Later in childhood, the level eases off before increasing with age among adults. More than half of all prescriptions for sleeping medicine are issued to patients aged over sixty-five. Women also appear more vulnerable than men: around 1.3 times more women than men report sleep difficulties.

IV

On my way out of the house one morning I bump into an old acquaintance from my youth; he's standing halfway out in the road in front of my building hooking up a trailer of cement sacks when I recognise him. We give each other a quick update: he's handling a drainage job for my neighbour; I tell him about the book I'm writing.

'Sleeplessness?' He lets go of the trailer hitch and points a finger at his own chest.

'I've struggled with it for years.'

When I tell people I don't sleep, their first reaction isn't shock or pity – instead I get to hear about other people who sleep badly: a friend, a wife, a son, a colleague. Or they suffer themselves.

This new openness about my sleep difficulties hasn't helped my nightly sleep but it has given me a long list of *other* insomniacs. It gradually dawns on me that it's no good just collecting names; I have to try and find out who these other sleepless people really are.

Inevitably, I have some reservations: everybody complains about their sleep, after all. I've got used to sleep deprivation so a night of just three hours' sleep is fine for me, whereas 'only' seven hours' sleep in a night can be a nightmare for others. It's difficult to distinguish between a person with insomnia and one who sleeps badly now and then. Fortunately, some diagnostic criteria have been established for insomnia. Sleep scientists agreed on them as recently as 2014.[46]

Before the diagnosis of insomnia is assigned, other causes must be ruled out. If people are ill or in severe pain, it isn't easy to get a good night's sleep. Chronic muscle pain can lead to a mixture of rapid and slow brain activity during deep sleep. Delta sleep doesn't work properly and the patient wakes up less rested. Metabolic diseases result in less deep sleep; frequent urination and nocturnal asthma attacks are other obvious causes. Sleep difficulties with such external causes are known as *secondary* insomnia.

A few people have what is known as *idiopathic* insomnia, which starts early, often in childhood. These are sleep problems that do not alter in response to factors in the person's life such as stress and anxiety – the person sleeps badly no matter what they do. Idiopathic quite simply means *without cause*. The disorder is assumed to result from deficient neural control over the parts of the brain that control sleeping and waking.

Some people suffer from *imagined* sleeplessness, which is an extreme variant of the self-deception we fall into when we believe we have slept much more poorly than we actually have. The sufferer of imagined sleeplessness feels that he or she is not sleeping enough despite getting enough sleep. They remember the wakeful periods in the night but fail to register the sleep. This is not merely a nocturnal experience: the next day they feel worn out and tired. It can be difficult to get to the bottom of it. So this condition can only be confirmed through a sleep study known as polysomnography – a lie detector for sleep, if you will.

And then there are those lucky people who simply don't require the same amount of sleep as the rest of us, but just haven't realised it themselves. When they wake up at 4 a.m. feeling refreshed they think something is wrong.

If we ignore these variants of sleeplessness, we're left with the most common form of insomnia: *psychophysiological* insomnia or learned sleeplessness. As the term suggests, the cause lies with the insomniacs themselves. Certain criteria must be met for this diagnosis to apply: first of all the most obvious one – you must lie awake at night. The most common thing is for it to take a long time to fall asleep. You lie there but sleep does not come. Waking up in the middle of the night and being unable to go back to sleep is another variant. And, finally, waking up early. A thirty-minute limit generally applies. If you take longer than that to fall asleep, lie awake for longer than that during the night or wake half an hour too early, those are signs of insomnia.

The sleepless person's subjective experience is not simply crucial to the diagnosis; it is the only thing available to relate to. The sleepless person must feel that their condition leads to diminished functioning during the day. In other words, sleeplessness is defined just as much by the day as the night. The sleep deprivation must be significant enough to be noticeable, in the form of tiredness, diminished capacity to spend time with other people, to perform one's job, to remember and concentrate – to function, in short. We may sleep a little or lightly during the night, but if we have no problems during the daytime, we have nonetheless got all the sleep we need.

One bad night is not enough, either. The sleep difficulties must be of a certain scope and a certain duration. If you have slept poorly for at least three nights a week for over a month, you may have short-term insomnia. If it continues for a further three months – welcome to the club: you have chronic insomnia.

'Think of a time when you closed the lid of a laptop to put it to sleep, but came back later to find that the screen was still on, the cooling fans were running and the computer was still active, despite the closed lid. Normally, this is because the programs and routines are still running, and the machine cannot make the transition into sleep mode.'[47] This is how Walker describes insomnia. In other words, sleeplessness is not simply an absence of the processes that make us fall asleep, and sleep deeply and continuously; things *happening* in the body and brain are keeping us awake. The body's fight-or-flight mechanism has helped humans to survive various threats throughout history. Normally, it's supposed to be activated when we are in danger and deactivated once the danger is past. But in many people suffering from insomnia, this mechanism is overactive. They are easily worried, cannot free themselves of the thought that some danger is imminent, that something terrible will happen. In this state, we are prepared to fight or flee, but in no condition to fall asleep, let alone sleep well and long.

Walker writes:

First, the raised metabolic rate triggered by fight-or-flight nervous system activity, which is common in insomnia patients, results in a higher core body temperature […] Second are higher levels of the alertness-promoting

112

hormone cortisol, and sister neurochemicals adrenaline and noradrenaline. All three of these chemicals raise heart rate. Normally our cardiovascular system calms down as we make the transition into light and then deep sleep. Elevated cardiac activity makes that transition more difficult. [...] third, and related to these chemicals, are altered patterns of brain activity [...] Recursive loops of emotional programs, together with retrospective and prospective memory loops, keep playing in the mind, preventing the brain from shutting down and switching into sleep mode. It is telling that a direct and causal connection exists between the fight and flight branch of the nervous system and all of these emotion-, memory-, and alertness-related regions of the brain. The bidirectional line of communication between the body and brain amounts to a vicious, recurring cycle that fuels their thwarting of sleep. The fourth and final set of identified changes has been observed in the quality of sleep of insomnia patients when they do finally drift off. Once again, these appear to have their origins in an overactive fight-or-flight nervous system. Patients with insomnia have a lower quality of sleep, reflected in shallower, less powerful electrical brainwaves during deep NREM [not REM sleep]. They also have more fragmented REM sleep, peppered by brief awakenings that they are not always aware of, yet still cause a degraded quality of dream sleep. All of which means that insomnia patients wake up not feeling refreshed.[48]

V

Two weeks after my meeting with Njål, I padlock my bike outside the coffee shop in Sagene and go inside to meet yet another insomniac – this time a stranger. She's a friend of a friend of Line's whom I've never met; all I know is that her name is Ingrid and she doesn't sleep at night.

I let my glance slide over the café but can't see anybody who seems to be waiting for me. Big windows, high ceilings, pale-brown cement floor and bare pale-brown walls. On the occasions I've been here with the kids early in the morning on weekends, it has been empty, but now there are people sitting at all the tables. It must be the lunchtime rush, or maybe not – most of them seem to be working on something, generally in pairs, with laptops and notebooks between them.

According to the philosopher and religious historian Roger Schmidt, sleeplessness emerged as a modern problem at the same time as places like this: cafés or coffee houses in London.[49] Before that, during the Renaissance, sleep was a virtue, something to strive for – *the poor man's wealth*, as the poet Sir Philip Sidney put it.

> *Come Sleep! O sleep, the certain knot of peace,*
> *The bathing place of wit, the balm of woe,*
> *The poor man's wealth, the prisoner's release,*
> *Th'indifferent judge between the high and low.*

But, writes Schmidt, all this started to change in the 1600s. In the West, sleep increasingly came to be seen as a waste of time and idleness, while being up and squeezing as many waking hours as possible into the day became the ideal. Time is money, as the insomniac Benjamin Franklin wrote in 1748. What happened to sleep in the time between Sidney's poem and Franklin's maxim? What made us stop seeing sleep as a boon and start treating it as a necessary evil?

Schmidt highlights some important innovations of the Enlightenment era. In London in around 1650 ever-increasing numbers of tea and coffee houses were set up. These two drinks rapidly became popular, first among the British and later among other Western Europeans – initially because of their ability to ward off sleepiness. Another new habit Londoners acquired was reading. The 1600s also gave us the novel, which made prolonged reading more enjoyable and accessible. It became common to read in bed, often late into the night – an activity often accompanied by copious cups of coffee or tea. Humanity's relationship with time also altered with the introduction of the pocket watch in the latter half of the 1600s. Being able to put time in one's own pocket is surely one of the greatest steps humanity has taken away from the state of nature. Time became individualised and people liberated themselves from the earthbound circadian rhythm. When they wondered what time of the day it was, they went from looking up at the sky to looking down into the palm of their own hand. The sense of time humanity bore within it before the pocket watch must have dissipated gradually. Humanity gained greater control over time, but it was, simultaneously, as if time and humanity parted ways.

Coffee, reading and the pocket watch lifted humanity out of the natural tides of sleep, bearing us further inland, where we gained greater control over our waking hours. Humans ceased to be creatures who let sleep come and go on its own terms and started to deny themselves the rest they needed. We liberated ourselves from nightly sleep – or so we thought, at least.

Samuel Johnson, of the eponymous dictionary, was one of many to embrace the new age and shun sleep:

Short, O short then be thy reign, and give us to the world again! ran his protest song against sleep.

With all these enlightened people sitting up late at night, increasing numbers of people were tired during the day. It became more common to lie in until midday. Schmidt thinks the change in Western people's sleeping patterns even affected furniture design: before 1660, all European chairs were constructed with a ninety-degree angle between seat and back. The chair was for sitting on, not relaxing in. But gradually, as night-time sleep diminished daytime weariness grew, and people sought ways to rest during the day. Items of furniture such as wing chairs saw the light of day in around 1700 and were designed to enable people to take a nap without being discovered while keeping their wigs on. The design has remained almost unchanged in the intervening three hundred years.

A woman in her thirties comes through the door and looks around. That must be her, so I get up, go over and say her name. Ingrid smiles and reaches out a hand, and I think that she *looks* like a person who doesn't sleep at night. Not that she looks tired or unrested, no – it's just something in her manner. A quiet restlessness, a sensitivity. Here's a person who likes coffee and books. A person like Samuel Johnson and me. We sit down, each with a coffee, black. Her dialect is from somewhere in the northern county of Trøndelag.

Sleep is a private thing, I think. Sleep is humanity at its most withdrawn and susceptible. A failure as fundamental as this, being unable to sleep, leaves one even more vulnerable. And then there is the constant thought I cannot rid myself of after all these years. *Why* can't she sleep? By asking about sleep, am I pouring salt on one of Ingrid's most painful, most open wounds? For sixteen years, I have kept my sleep problems to myself and now I expect this person I have never met before to tell me about hers? What do I really hope to achieve with this conversation?

What I need is somebody who actually understands. Doctors, authors of self-help books, acupuncturists, yoga teachers – what do they know about not sleeping? About being so tired that your own feet trip you up on the pavement? About having slept so little that you think you see things creeping around at the edges of your vision? About being so desperate over your lack of night-time peace that you burst out crying when a faulty battery sets the smoke alarm beeping in the middle of the night? After all, this isn't like a disease or an injury, where there's a fixed point on the body you can focus your gaze on and battle against. Insomnia is like a sackful of symptoms I'm carrying around, and every time I see a new person, they pull a diagnosis out of the sack that best fits their own understanding of the world. And all these people I'm opening up to – family, friends, acquaintances – none of them understand what I'm showing them, either; they can never understand. They may listen to me, feel sorry for me, advise me to paint my bedroom walls blue, but every night they lie in their beds and sleep long and deep until the next morning.

After some niceties, we fall silent and I decide to dive in. I put down my cup of coffee.

'How did you sleep last night?'

SEPTEMBER

Murder and Other Sleep Difficulties

About witches, crocodiles and other creatures that can appear when you think you are awake; and about how sleepwalking can be the best defence against a murder charge.

I

Summer is over. I'm sleeping better at night but that doesn't mean I'm cured. The new pattern: every night I go to bed at the normal time, before midnight. I doze off or fall into something resembling sleep. Then I wake up an hour later. I get out of bed and go up to the TV room where I settle on the sofa and put on a film; and there, sometime between one and three in the morning, I fall into a deep sleep and sleep soundly until I'm woken by the rest of the family. For the first few minutes I'm like a newly hatched chick hauled up out of my deep, protective sleep, dazed and warm, and I want only to return to the delicious darkness. Slowly I get moving, preparing packed lunches, dressing the kids, downing the first cup of coffee. My battery is fully charged and will see me through the whole day. Strong, rested, fully functioning until night comes and the whole process repeats itself.

Everything is better as long as I get sleep. I am more productive, write more and better. I perform better at work. Every task, from picking detritus up from the living room floor to clearing out the storeroom in the cellar, seems unproblematic. My family gets a better version of me. It's as if somebody has switched on a lamp, allowing me to see all the things I have in life: a wife, two children, the ability and opportunity to write books, produce comic strips and make music; a career, a place to live.

But then I get home from work and see the blanket and pillows on the sofa, the place where I spend my nights. A person incapable of sleeping in his own bed is not a functional person.

Yet still I continue to lie on the sofa, every night, because I know it works. One night when Line is away on a work trip, I spend the whole day looking forward to the night because I won't have to take anybody else into account: I can go straight to the sofa, get even more sleep without having to spend that first, pointless hour in bed.

Have I given up?

I'm back where I was many years ago, after the previous round of trying different treatment methods. Everything repeats itself – this too. On that occasion I also exhausted the possibilities out there and started seeking them at home. The only place I finally found sleep was on the floor in front of the TV. A pillow, a blanket, directly on the wooden floor. At least now I lie on a piece of furniture. But the sofa is like methadone: it isn't a lasting solution. Not just because it isn't socially acceptable to spend your nights on the sofa when you have a bed and a partner to share it with. Line jokes about it, saying that since the bedroom only belongs to her – just like her own childhood bedroom – she may as well hang up posters of Alice Cooper on the walls. But I know that she, like me, finds it sad that although we go to bed together, I end up elsewhere during the night. I also know this isn't something I can keep doing over the long term. The moment my brain accepts the sofa as the approved sleeping spot, I won't be able to sleep there either. To sleep on the sofa is to give way to irrationality. Because I'm alone and it happens at night, I can let my own self-contradictory mind have its way, with no consequences for anybody but myself. If I did it by daylight, in front of other people, I'd long ago have been branded a nervous wreck.

I try to explain the sofa situation to Ingrid the next time we meet to exchange experiences.

'It works as long as I know I'm *not* supposed to be sleeping there,' I say.

'You should move the sofa into your bedroom,' she says.

For three weeks, Ingrid has slept poorly, she tells me. Her pattern resembles my own. She wakes at the same time every night, 1.50 a.m., and can't get back to sleep. And she is incapable of lying in the same bed as her boyfriend, who falls asleep in an instant and always sleeps the whole night through.

'He sleeps and I'm left lying awake. I think about how desperately in need of sleep I am and it just doesn't happen. I lie there watching the clock as it turns three then four then five o'clock. At six o'clock I generally get up and leave for work.'

'That's the worst thing you can do, clock-watch,' I say. 'But you know that, of course.'

'Just now, I'm worn so ragged that I can't control myself, I just can't manage it. Nothing seems to go right. At work, I have a really short fuse and I get so clumsy I can't even formulate a text message. When I get home in the afternoons, I'm totally wiped out. I should exercise or go for a walk, but I can't be bothered. Can't even manage to walk to and from work because my body is so sluggish. And when I pass the intersection on Carl Berner I have to block my ears because I can't cope with all the traffic noise.'

'The worst thing is those lorries with empty truck beds and heavy, dangling chains – when they drive past at full speed and their chains rattle on the bends, I'm terrified the whole thing is going to tip over on top of me,' I say.

'I remember this one incident,' Ingrid continues. 'My boyfriend and I walked past a woman begging with a cup outside the Oslo City shopping centre. She walked up to another couple walking ahead of us on the pavement and they just shoved her aside, as if they were shooing away a pigeon. It was so aggressive and awful and it shook me to the core. I had no filter. I got so upset. At the same time, I didn't manage to say anything. It coloured the rest of our day. And then my boyfriend got angry with me because I couldn't pull myself together and I let it ruin things for both of us. Everything went off the rails and in the end we had to go home. If I'd slept, I would have coped with it. Oh, I'm so tired of saying *I slept badly!*'

Ingrid tells me she's turned down an invitation to a confirmation this weekend because of her sleeplessness and the bad patch she's currently going through.

'I should be there but I just can't deal with all the people. You expend so much energy on just being nice. But I get a bit cross with myself too. How difficult can it be? After all, I could just sit in a corner chatting with Grandma.'

Ingrid doesn't have a before and after, either – she's struggled with sleep ever since she was a baby, according to her mother, and throughout the whole of her childhood. In her teens she slept a lot, but as an adult she's never slept more than five or six hours in a row. She's been through two rounds of psychotherapy without any success, and otherwise resorts to yoga, nocturnal walks and podcasts. And *Gilmore Girls* and chess tournaments on TV, which calm her down, she says.

'How does it feel when you sleep well?' I ask.

'Every time I'm rested, I think: is this how it feels? I'm brimming over with energy, almost euphoric. I make masses of arrangements with people and sort out everything I've been putting off. I hang pictures on the wall. It's no effort at all. I'm always disappointed when the good patch ends and the sleeplessness returns.'

Before we part, Ingrid tells me about another sleep-related experience that makes my hair stand on end:

'I'm lying in bed with my face turned to the wall. Suddenly I realise there's somebody in the room behind me. I can't turn around. The presence comes closer and then I feel somebody lying down beside me, partly on top of me. I feel their weight in the bed. I'm scared to death but still can't turn around. Then I see a hand, a female hand, descend in front of my face. I catch a glimpse of a nightdress and long fair hair. Then it vanishes and I can move again.'

'God almighty! What did you do?'

'I packed a bag and moved in with my brother.'

Experiences like this are known as *hypnagogic hallucinations*, where dream activity begins before we have managed to fall asleep, or *hypnopompic hallucinations*, where it continues after sleep but before we are properly awake. The dreams bleed into our conscious mind. We may see and hear things that do not exist – people or terrifying creatures in the bedroom or the ceiling breaking up into colourful patterns above our bed and so on. Oliver Sacks devoted a section to this phenomenon in his book *Hallucinations*, detailing examples given by a man who suffered from hypnopompic hallucinations: 'A huge figure of an angel standing over me next to a figure of death in black.' 'A rotting corpse lying next to me.' 'A huge crocodile at my throat'.[50] It isn't unusual for patients with this disorder to be reluctant to tell others about it for fear of being seen as mad. In some cases, like Ingrid's, the hallucinations are accompanied by a temporary inability to move. This is called *sleep paralysis*. The muscular paralysis of the REM stage persists even though we are fully conscious and have managed to open our eyes. In the worst cases, we may lie as if shackled to our bed, unable to move as gruesome sights and sounds play out in our bedroom.

Dreams that have crossed the boundary between the waking and sleeping state have inspired humanity in various ways throughout history. Henry Fuseli's famous, terrifying painting *The Nightmare* from 1781 and Eugène Thivier's sculpture *Cauchemar* from 1894 both represent the experience of sleep paralysis. Fritz Schwimbeck's drawing *Mein Traum, Mein Böser Traum* from 1915 is, perhaps, the most fearsome depiction of sleep paralysis. Rodney Ascher's horror documentary, *The Nightmare* (2015), gives us an insight into how gruesome the experiences during sleep paralysis can be. The most unsettling thing is that a great many of the people interviewed in the film have had similar visions: shadow men, the hat man, the old witch, extraterrestrial-like figures, the cat on their chest, glowing red eyes in the dark. A friend of mine who has experienced episodes of sleep paralysis describes almost exactly the same thing: a kind of shadow man standing over him saying, *your soul belongs to me*. Some people even think that sleep paralysis is the origin of most superstitions and conspiracy theories. Ghosts, aliens, monsters... were they all – as the compositions I wrote at school inevitably used to conclude – just a dream?

But if they are dreams, why do we all dream the same thing?

Midnight. The others are asleep; the silence is broken only by creakings from our upstairs neighbours and whimpers from the kids downstairs. I shower, and butter a couple of slices of bread. Normally I relish this time of day. This is when, sleepless or not, I have a chance to recover and seek peace before night comes. But now I look over my shoulder in the shower, and when I go from the kitchen to the TV room, I creep along the walls. I can't stop thinking about *her*, the woman in Ingrid's hallucination. I love being scared, but in a controlled, predictable form – an H. P. Lovecraft story, say, or a Dario Argento film. Something I can seek out and abandon whenever I choose. The thought that an experience like Ingrid's could happen at any time scares me out of my wits. The idea that somebody could suddenly *be standing there in front of me*, or come sneaking up behind me – while I'm incapable of movement. Could anything be worse? Sleep paralysis isn't associated with insomnia, or not as far as I know at any rate. But if it's happened to Ingrid, it could happen to me too.

I sit down on the sofa, back to the corner so that I have an overview of the room, and feel my heart pounding. I believe in science, shun anything based on conviction, but in the grip of my fear I'm inclined to believe anything at all. I left my glass of milk in the kitchen but I daren't go back and fetch it now.

Dare I sleep?

II

I get an e-mail with a blue link from a pal. *Have you seen this?* he asks. Over recent months, I've been getting increasing numbers of e-mails like this from friends: internet links about insomnia. I've become the sleepless guy. Usually, they're articles with the usual tips about remembering to keep your bedroom cool, setting aside an hour for your worries before going to bed and so on.

This link takes me to a *Guardian* article. The title 'Finally, a cure for insomnia?' doesn't exactly set my pulse racing. On the contrary, given my experience over recent months, the sight of a sentence combining the words *sleeplessness* and *cure* arouses nothing but suspicion. But the text is published in a reputable British newspaper and written by a journalist who suffers from insomnia himself. So I read it.

It's about The Insomnia Clinic in London, which has revolutionised the treatment of sleeplessness in the United Kingdom. Eighty per cent of the patients experience a significant improvement in their sleep difficulties, while half say they are completely cured. The clinic was set up in 2009 by a South African psychiatrist and former insomniac, Hugh Selsick. When Selsick started working as a psychiatrist at the end of the nineties, he discovered that nobody was treating insomnia, even though sleeplessness was extremely widespread among patients with mental health problems. Psychiatry didn't take on patients with insomnia, and centres dealing with sleep difficulties only studied issues such as snoring and breathing problems.

Insomnia, the journalist writes, has been the 'Cinderella of medicine' for several decades.

The treatment Selsick has developed consists of a five-week programme that combines cognitive behavioural therapy and sleep efficiency training.

Cognitive therapy, I think; that was what I tried many years ago, and it was both expensive and disappointing. And sleep efficiency training – didn't Njål talk about something like that?

There's something familiar about the description of the clinic and the treatment. I search around until I find a Norwegian newspaper article I read earlier, a story about people struggling to sleep at night. In the end, I find what I'm looking for. 'Here at Lovisenberg Diakonale Hospital they study sleep problems and assign diagnoses,' it reads, below a photograph of two people in white coats.[51] I look at the photograph of the pair, captioned *Sleep doctors* – in the foreground an older man wearing glasses who is waving his arms in the air enthusiastically while a younger woman sits by a PC listening to him.

Is this a Norwegian variant of Selsick's clinic?

I ring the hospital's contact centre. I tell the woman at the other end of the line that I have insomnia; is it possible to make contact with the people who were interviewed in the article? She asks whether I'm ringing for an interview or for treatment. I go quiet, realising that I don't exactly know what I want. Yes, please – both?

'I went to my GP and got a referral,' I say.

'To the Sleep School?'

'No, to a sleep study at the sleep laboratory. But the referral was rejected.'

'Well, I don't think you need a sleep study if you suffer from insomnia,' the woman says hesitantly, as if addressing an innocent child she wishes to shield from the brutal truth. 'Sleep studies are for physiological problems, like sleep apnoea, that kind of thing. You can talk to one of the people who runs courses for patients with insomnia here at our place. They're psychologists.'

Afterwards I look up the various courses offered on the hospital's website. *Better Self-Esteem, Dealing with Depression, The Art of Saying No, Help, I Eat too Much!, Dealing with Social Anxiety*. At the bottom of the list are details of the Sleep School. 'The Sleep School builds on knowledge of good sleeping habits and cognitive theory. The participants will be trained in cognitive models to alter their own inappropriate thoughts and patterns of behaviour associated with their sleep problems. On the course the participants will learn more about what sleep is, what perpetuates bad sleeping habits and what it takes to alter them. Sleep restriction is a central part of this course and will often demand a high level of motivation and personal effort from the participants.'

After reading the two articles and talking to the hospital's communications officer, I am both disappointed and relieved. Disappointed because I realise that I haven't advanced a single step in the past six months. Relieved because I now spy a possible treatment that appears to be accepted in established medical circles.

But first and foremost I am puzzled. Where does my insomnia belong? As a child I suffered from appendicitis: after I'd lain there for several days writhing from the stomach pains, Grandad rang A&E and in a mere two hours I was taken to hospital, anaesthetised and operated on. A year later, I suffered from volvulus and received the same rapid, appropriate treatment. At Ålesund Hospital there was even a dedicated department for my problem, with specialist doctors and nurses.

But when I develop insomnia twenty years later, nobody knows where I should turn. I become the

Cinderella of medicine and don't belong anywhere, which means I belong everywhere – so I go to anybody who will have me: psychiatrists, yoga teachers, acupuncturists, meditation centres, anybody who can offer friendly advice. I eat bananas before bedtime, take a hot shower after midnight, download apps that promise to soothe my mind and send me to sleep; I've become well versed in the world of tea and I've even *moved house* in order to sleep better. I have made myself a new life, become a different person in my efforts to get sleep.

And now I've spent half a year waiting for a sleep study before being rejected. Why have I been so passive? Because I've felt the need for *something*, something to hope for, I've avoided looking into what this kind of study would actually involve and whether it would even help me.

'I don't understand a thing any more,' I say to Line. 'Should I do a sleep study or go to therapy? My GP doesn't seem to have a clue and I can't be guided by these newspaper articles either. I have to talk to a scientist. Somebody who has acquired knowledge about sleep and sleeping disorders and doesn't just offer theories and treatment methods based on their own perception of reality.'

'You have to be patient,' says Line, who's a journalist and experienced in trying to get hold of people from every conceivable walk of life. 'Sleep scientists are the busiest people in the world.'

'They work with *sleep*,' I say. 'How busy can they be?'

III

Nature seems to have found every possible variant of divergence from the norm of lying quietly in your bed

and sleeping. Previously I haven't been all that interested in sleep problems other than my own, and didn't
believe there was anything other than insomnia. Now,
after reading how fragile the sleeping state is and how
much can happen before, during and after sleep, I find
it even more incredible that anybody ever sleeps at all.

There are currently more than a hundred different
diagnoses for different sleep disorders, the majority of
which fall into four categories: hypersomnia, circadian
rhythm disorders, parasomnia and insomnia. Within
these groups, we find everything from minor disorders to
serious diseases that make it impossible to lead a normal
life – everything from small, unnoticeable symptoms in
the darkness of the night to the most hysterical episodes.

Hypersomnia involves an increased need for sleep
and, now and then, spells of daytime sleeping. *Hyper* is
Latin for *over* or *too much*. These are chronic diseases the
sufferer must generally have had for at least six months
in order to be assigned a diagnosis.

The 'most minor' cases of hypersomnia may have
causes as simple as snoring or sleep-disordered
breathing. Half of all adult humans snore. Snoring is
caused by the vibrations of the breath as it passes the
roof of the mouth and the uvula. Sometimes it causes
a loud noise, other times the noise is less of a problem.
Snoring can be a nuisance for the person lying beside the
snorer who is trying to sleep, and it can also curtail the
snorer's own sleep.

Sleep-disordered breathing, also known as sleep
apnoea, is more troublesome. Apnoea is a Greek
word that means 'no air.' Parts of the airways that
vibrate during snoring collapse, which happens more
frequently in REM sleep than in the other stages.
Sleep-disordered breathing can last for anything from

ten seconds to more than a minute and many episodes may occur in a single night. Needless to say, this leads to tiredness in the day. Sleep apnoea mostly affects men and the most common cause is being overweight. Pickwickian Syndrome – breathing difficulties affecting overweight people that lead, among other things, to constant daytime tiredness – is named after a character in Dickens's *The Pickwick Papers*: an overweight serving boy who falls asleep at every possible opportunity throughout the day. Treatments for these disorders can be as simple as losing weight or cutting out alcohol, pills and cigarettes. Some sufferers have to sleep wearing a mask that supplies oxygen at a high enough pressure to prevent their airways from collapsing. In some cases, people may undergo a surgical procedure.

The other type of hypersomnia is associated with the central nervous system and is known as narcolepsy. This involves abnormal sleepiness and episodes of daytime sleeping. People can quite simply be ambushed by sleep at any moment. In the film *My Own Private Idaho*, the main character played by River Phoenix suffers from this condition. He falls asleep in the most unlikely situations throughout the day. The disease is rare, affecting fewer than one per cent of the population. Most people with narcolepsy also develop cataplexy, a temporary loss of muscular strength sparked by abrupt emotional triggers. Fits of laughter, a shock, anger, stress or physical exertion can all cause a sudden loss of power in large or small parts of the victim's musculature, causing them to collapse while remaining aware of their surroundings. These episodes usually pass after a few minutes.

Not to be confused with cataplexy is an altogether more disturbing condition: catalepsy, which results in muscular rigidity and decreased sensitivity to pain. The sufferer may sink into a deathlike state, which has made this condition a popular subject for literature and film, especially in the horror and crime genres. It is easy to see why the phenomenon would appeal to writers keen to come up with new ways of tricking their readers: everyone around you is convinced you are dead and yet you are still alive. Edgar Allan Poe knew a great deal about this disease, most probably because of his own fear of being buried in a state where he would be able to experience it happening but would be incapable of stopping it. He devoted space to it in several of his works, including the short story *The Premature Burial*: 'Sometimes, without any apparent cause, I sank, little by little, into a condition of hemi-syncope, or half swoon; and, in this condition, without pain, without ability to stir, or, strictly speaking, to think, but with a dull lethargic consciousness of life and of the presence of those who surrounded my bed, I remained, until the crisis of the disease restored me, suddenly, to perfect sensation.'

Catalepsy, as depicted in 19th century literature, no longer exists, or not in the medical world at any rate. Perhaps it was simply one of those exaggerations of the Victorian era – like so much else – because now it occurs only in short episodes that are over before anybody has a chance to call the undertakers.

But catalepsy does not belong among the sleep disorders, unlike cataplexy. One theory holds that cataplexy is REM sleep gone wrong; that this stage of sleep blends with the waking state, and that the suspension of muscular activity is the same process that occurs during REM sleep.

Circadian rhythm disorders involve a reduced capacity or ability to maintain a regular rhythm. Some people live without a circadian rhythm, others have a fluid cycle in which their nightly sleep shifts several hours over every cycle, so that they experience every possible variant of circadian rhythm over the course of a couple of weeks. Blind people may experience problems with circadian rhythm because those isolated from the sight of light are also isolated from its regulating effect. In such cases, people have to compensate by finding other ways to draw a clear distinction between night and day, with the help of a regular wake-up time, fixed mealtimes and, in some cases, intake of melatonin. Delayed sleep phase syndrome, where people sleep and wake later than usual, affects people most often in puberty and their early twenties. Although it may sound like the bad habits of lazy teenagers who enjoy staying up late at night, this is actually a genetic disorder. The internal clock – which should normally be set for a cycle of roughly twenty-four hours and fifteen minutes – may be set for longer than that – in some cases as long as forty hours[52], so almost the same circadian rhythm as the Somali cavefish! Circadian rhythm disorders in humans may be corrected through light therapy, which generally involves blocking blue light at night and using a bright light lamp early in the morning. This disorder can also go the opposite way: advanced deep phase syndrome is where people fall asleep early in the evening and wake up in the middle of the night. It's the same condition in reverse but is treated much more rarely. A circadian rhythm that involves going to bed early and getting up at dawn isn't just easier to adapt to a normal working life; it is socially acceptable and even seen by some as a virtue. This illustrates a fundamental trait of several of the sleeping disorders and especially circadian rhythm disorders. They are not always damaging to the health or a nuisance in themselves; the problem is the pressure to adapt to other people. As humans, we have no need for regularity in isolation. Shifting our circadian rhythm or staying awake through the night won't make us ill, as long as we sleep at some point. The issue here is sleeping and waking when others sleep and wake.

Parasomnia is a term that covers unusual activities during sleep. This is the category in which we find the most eventful sleep problems. As a rule they pass of their own accord and are not directly damaging to the health – although in special circumstances they may pose a danger to both the sleeper and other people.

Many of the disorders are associated with the transition between the sleeping and waking states, like the best known example: sleepwalking. Like many of the other parasomnias, sleepwalking – somnambulism – occurs because the different stages of sleep get mixed up. Sleepwalking generally happens in the first part of the night when the sleeper is making the transition from deep sleep into lighter sleep. Instead of waking up, the sleepwalker has an incomplete awakening – a hybrid stage that combines elements of both deep sleep and wakefulness. Sleepwalking is commonest among children, most frequently those aged five to twelve[53]. From 15 to 30 per cent of all healthy children walk in their sleep now and then, while 3 per cent of all healthy children walk in their sleep frequently. Infants may sleepwalk while in bed but their parents won't always find out, often because the bars or high edges of the cot prevent the child from actually going anywhere.

A child who has got out of bed and onto their feet will normally wander round quietly and calmly, without major incident. Children often walk towards light sources or their parents' bed, and may urinate just beside the toilet or in the corner of the room. Parents with children who sleepwalk may wake to find the child standing by their bedside. As a rule the girl or boy allows themselves to be led back to their own bed. Their eyes are open and glazed. Does the child see anything? Does he or she take in sights and sounds? If so, everything is forgotten the next day.

Only 1 per cent of adults are sleepwalkers. Most of those who sleepwalk also have family members who do or have done it. An episode of somnambulism can last from five minutes to around half an hour. It is normal to walk in your sleep when you are sleeping most deeply and are most difficult to wake. Although it is a myth that it is harmful for sleepwalkers to be woken up, it can be hard to rouse them because they are in deep sleep, so confusion and dangerous situations can arise. Older children and adults can lapse into a state known as *agitated sleepwalking*, where the sleepwalker resists efforts to lead them back to bed or be woken up. They behave more wildly than the more biddable small children – lamps are overturned, some try to walk through glass doors and others even leave the house.

What might make somebody get out of bed and start wandering around in their sleep? Noises, light or something as simple as having a full bladder. Factors that can contribute to increasing the share of deep sleep, such as sleep deprivation, exhaustion and stress, can also trigger somnabulism. Bullying may be one of the factors that triggers sleepwalking in children.

Another variant of parasomnia is *confused awakening*, a condition that can arise if a person is abruptly woken up from the first deep stages of sleep, generally early in the night. The person wakes up yet doesn't wake up, doesn't respond to questions and quite simply behaves strangely: they may talk incoherently and some may become angry. The confused awakening may last anything from a few minutes to several hours. Later the person remembers nothing.

Incubus, also known as night terror, is an abrupt awakening from the deep stages of sleep during the first three hours of the night. The term refers to a male demon believed in Medieval times to seduce women at night. A night terror generally starts with a shriek. The victim displays all the signs of genuine terror: dilated pupils, sweating, a high pulse rate and rapid breathing. Adults who suffer such night terrors may also be struggling with mental problems such as phobias, depression or anxiety. Among children, who are most commonly affected, the cause may be an immature central nervous system. But here, too, stress caused by, say, bullying may be the trigger. Night terrors are short in duration and people rarely remember them afterwards, in contrast to the baby brother of the night terror, the nightmare.

It may sound odd to call bad dreams a sleeping disorder. We've all had bad dreams, after all. Unlike night terrors, nightmares generally occur in the last REM stages of night-time sleep and are dreams so unpleasant that they wake us up. Why some people are haunted by nightmares is unclear – but among adults who are frequently affected, more suffer mental health problems than not. Some studies suggest that people who often have nightmares may be more sensitive, with a better developed imagination.[54]

The type of parasomnia known as RBD, or *REM sleep behaviour disorder*, is a sleeping disorder in which people have violent dreams without the paralysis that normally accompanies REM sleep. In other words, those affected live out their dreams in reality as they sleep. Hitting, kicking, running, shouting and laughter manifest as violent thrashing in the bed, and it isn't unusual in such cases for the sleeper to injure their bed partner. RBD almost exclusively affects older men.

Other parasomnic phenomena, such as talking or grinding your teeth in your sleep or hypnic jerks – those violent starts we may experience on the edge of sleep – are things all of us may be affected by or experience through the people with whom we share our bed. There is even one form of parasomnia that sounds like something straight out of *The Exorcist*: head-rolling or -banging, or a rhythmic rocking of the body as the person kneels up in bed on all fours. Or episodes where the sleeper has sex without waking up: sexsomnia – or, as some call it, snoregasm. This is not the same as a wet dream, which is not classified as a sleep disorder.

Parasomnic episodes may seem dramatic but they are almost always harmless. Only rarely do things go too far, as in the case of Ken Parks.[55] In 1987, this American was charged with the murder of his mother-in-law and the attempted murder of his father-in-law. There was no doubt that he had carried out the act: Parks had left his own home late at night, driven twenty-three kilometres, entered his parents-in-law's house, attacked his mother-in-law with a knife and then hit her on the head with a tyre iron. He had throttled his father-in-law until he lost consciousness.

An open-and-shut case of murder and attempted murder, right? A crime for which the vengeful American legal system would mete out the harshest possible punishment?

No.

According to Parks, he had done it all in his sleep. Afterwards, still sleeping, he had gone to the police station and turned himself in. When he was questioned later, he remembered nothing. Sleepwalking is not a defect, his defence ran during the trial, but a normal state in which the body acts without conscious signals to the brain. Consequently the sleepwalker cannot be held criminally responsible or deemed mentally ill. A neurologist vouched for this theory, that the accused was in a deep sleep from the moment he left home until the point when he turned himself in at the police station, and therefore could not be woken; the violence was most probably triggered by his mother-in-law's attempts to wake him. The car journey of more than *twenty kilometres* was also possible, according to the neurologist, because the eyes of the accused were open, and sleepwalkers are generally able to manoeuvre their way around their own home.

Parks was found innocent.

IV

After weeks of e-mailing, texting and telephoning, I still haven't succeeded in setting up a conversation with a sleep scientist. They are always on their way to some other part of the planet. *Leaving for China tomorrow. Try me in two weeks.* What is it with sleep scientists and all this travel? Where are they travelling to? Yet I daren't pester them too much, either; I'm afraid of disturbing them and have great respect for the work they do, which is, in many ways, trying to help people like me.

Finally, a sleep scientist calls me back – while I'm sitting in the bath, of course. I have no choice: I can't risk having to wait several more weeks for another chance, so I leap out of the bath, throw a dressing-gown around my wet body and take the call. Water drips off me and onto my notes as I try to explain to the sleep scientist what my situation is and what I want to talk to him about.

'I've had insomnia for sixteen years,' I start off. 'My doctor gave me sleeping pills but they don't help any more. So, he referred me for a sleep study, but I was rejected and in any case I'm pretty certain it wouldn't have helped.'

The sleep scientist sighs. His name is Børge Sivertsen and he is senior researcher at Norway's Public Health Institute.

'This is a major headache for those of us working on insomnia,' he says. 'We know how serious it is and we know the cost to society. And we do know – paradoxically enough – what it takes to treat insomnia. Yet the unfortunate fact is that sleeping pills prescribed by GPs are generally still the first option patients are offered. Sleeping pills can work, but they aren't a solution.'

'The Public Health Institute where you work has described sleep difficulties as one of the country's most underestimated public health problems. What do you mean by that?'

'It is underestimated because insomnia doesn't appear on the sickness absence statistics. We don't know what it costs society. There is no official diagnosis that gives people a right to sickness benefits. But we do know that mental illnesses such as anxiety and depression account for one-third of the social security budget, which amounts to billions of kroner a year. And we know that the risk of dropping out of the labour market is just as great for insomnia as for depression.'

At last, somebody who sees us, I think. Or at least our absence. A value has been assigned to my sleeplessness.

'What's more, we know that insomnia is on the rise in the Norwegian population,' Sivertsen continues. 'Most international studies show that around 10 per cent have such severe sleep difficulties that they fall into the category known as chronic insomnia. In Norway, we have seen a trend that diverges from the pattern elsewhere in the world in recent years – an increase from 10 to 15 per cent. We have become a slightly more sleepless people than before. We don't sleep less in terms of hours and minutes, but we are shifting our sleep-wake cycle and we sleep in a more fragmented way. We sleep at different times. We struggle to get enough good sleep, sleep a bit more lightly and we function more poorly in the daytime. In addition, we are seeing a marked increase in sleeplessness among young adults and young people in sixth form.'

'What's to blame?'

'We know that it's linked to the use of social media and electronic gadgets. The more time you spend in front of a screen or on a smartphone, the less time you sleep and the greater difficulty you have falling asleep. In the eighties, the TV was switched off after the evening news and then nothing else happened. The world is totally different now.'

'You said you know what it takes to treat insomnia,' I say.

'Yes,' Sivertsen says. 'The gold standard for treatment of insomnia…'

I stand over my desk writing notes, trying to keep the notebook and pen as far away from myself as possible to avoid dripping bathwater onto the pages. *Gold standard*, I write in red ink and wait for him to carry on. I feel my heart beating a little bit harder.

At last.

V

My GP gets up and shakes my hand as I come in. We smile and nod at one another like old friends. The gesture is warm and welcoming, a contrast to the attitude I am accustomed to from previous appointments, and for a moment I'm convinced that he knows me, knows everything about my insomnia and has come up with a solution he is now impatient to present to me. We sit down, he reaches for his mouse and fixes his gaze on the screen. I look around the doctor's surgery. One of those repulsive anatomical models showing a cross-section of a human abdomen – purple liver, pink kidneys, yellow stomach and gut – stands on a shelf of pale lacquered birch. Beside the door through which I just entered hang the doctor's outdoor clothes: a brown corduroy blazer and a big colourful scarf.

'Let's see,' the doctor says to the screen. 'Bortne.'

He's quiet for a while. Then he says, 'Insomnia,' with a semi-questioning tone in his voice as he looks at me.

'That's right,' I say, repressing an urge to add *the Cinderella of Medicine*.

He turns his gaze back to the screen. Then comes the ritual silence in which the doctor reads my notes. I sit still and wait as he looks at what he himself wrote about my last appointment, which was two-and-a-half months ago now. It's been five months since I first presented my problem and since that time, my sleepless existence has continued exactly as before: good nights, normal nights, bad nights, terrible nights. Since I sat in this chair five months ago, I have tried to conquer insomnia, to no avail. My sleep difficulties have simply persisted, inexorably, no matter what I have done. I'd have been better off not

140

even trying – at least then I could have used what little strength I had to recover. And since that time, the doctor has sat in this office, hanging his outdoor clothes on the hook by the door, calling in patients, reading through their notes and trying to find a solution for them. This young man, the locum of the locum of my GP seems like a professional, attentive and solicitous person but I am forgotten the instant I walk out of his office. Even before I've removed these idiotic orange plastic slippers, we're told to put on to protect the floor and stepped out into the autumn sunshine, he'll have moved on to the next patient. And then the next. And then the next. And 'Bortne, insomnia' will be nothing but an entry in my notes until next time I book an appointment.

A friend once said, 'If you want to get anywhere with the health system, you have to shout the same thing over and over again.' Without desperation, without headlines and exaggerations and endless repetitions and clear diagnoses and treatment alternatives you'll never manage to wake the doctors up from their trance. This is a job you have to do yourself.

It's my life, I'm the one lying awake at nights, I'm the one shuffling through the days, I'm the one being worn down, little by little; it's my family that has to cope with the exhaustion and personality changes of a person deprived of sleep. It's my career that's suffering. And it's my premature death this will lead to – if I'm to believe what the newspapers write about sleep deprivation. Just this morning I came across yet another news item, this time in an English newspaper, about a new study: mortality rates were 65 per cent higher for adults who slept five hours or fewer. Five hours! Five hours of continuous sleep is a victory for me! There should be a ban on writing articles like that.

My doctor has read my notes and now he looks at me.

'How can I help you?' he asks.

I show him the letter I received at the end of July, the rejection of my referral to a sleep study. That came more than two months ago now. I place the paper on the desk between us, like a prosecutor presenting proof. He cranes his neck and studies the document.

'My referral was rejected,' I say.

'Uh-huh?'

He picks up the letter and looks at it before handing it back to me and looking at his screen again, back at my notes.

'In the rejection letter, it says I have the right to request a new referral,' I say. It sounds as if I'm reading the rules straight off the lid of a board game, but it's true: You have the right to request one further assessment for the same condition, it says. *Take a card and roll the dice again*.

'I want a new referral. But I don't want to go for a sleep study, because that's no use.'

'No?'

'No.'

I get up and walk around the desk, stand behind the doctor and lean over, look at his screen.

'This is what I want you to write,' I say.

OCTOBER

Dark Time

About Facebook, LED light, how the world once lay
in darkness after sunset and the next generation of
insomniacs.

I

I like the first half of autumn: the sudden division
between day and night, the darkness that comes and
goes more swiftly, the temperature that dips lower
in the night. It's as if our part of the world seeks out
its original state. Everything becomes sharper – light,
colours, sounds. The features of passers-by seem more
distinct; the park smells of wet leaves. It's been a long
hot summer, but it's here in the quiet, dark cold that
we belong. For a few weeks, my sleep seems to behave
normally, maybe because my surroundings are normal
and therefore more sleep friendly. Light mornings, cool
days, dark evenings, chilly nights.

The last weekend in October, the clocks go back an
hour. I'm not bothered by this artificial shift in time. It
doesn't help my sleep, but it doesn't cause any disruption either. But it's worse for the kids, who get tired and
wake up at the same time every day throughout the
year. Some days they wake up at six o'clock; with this
new wintertime, they're now up at five o'clock. In the
evening they get tired earlier and we try to keep them

up for fifteen minutes extra until we've adjusted to the new rhythm.

Thanks, society.

A number of countries are currently reconsidering daylight saving. It was Benjamin Franklin who first mulled the idea of changing the clocks to exploit the daylight and thereby increase efficiency back in 1784. That's right, the time-is-money guy who was also a famous insomniac. In this respect, Franklin was a prototype of the irrational, destructive modern human: he battled sleeplessness by night and ruined the nightly sleep of his fellow men by day.

The thinking behind daylight saving is that putting the clocks forward an hour to ensure more daylight in the afternoons enables society to keep on doing whatever it is doing. In Franklin's day, that meant working in textile factories or building houses. Today, we can use the extra hour to style dogs, write blogs or devise communication strategies for senior executives who have done something untoward.

This shift comes at the expense of the mornings, affecting the point at which we are normally exposed to light for the first time in the day. A number of studies have shown that most people cope poorly with the transition to summertime.[56] The transition to wintertime, when the clocks go back an hour, is comparable to moving to a more westerly time zone. Since our inbuilt circadian rhythm involves a cycle of twenty-four hours and fifteen minutes, our body goes along with this shift – although we may suddenly feel the urge to get up and watch cartoons earlier than we'd like to. But when it goes the other way, when the clock is put forward an hour, it's equivalent to travelling to an easterly time zone – now you're working against nature and against the inbuilt rhythm, which wants to advance. A blow struck for society is a slap in the face for the individual. And sleep loses yet another swathe of its territory, set to flight by the new, efficient, waking world.

My friend Njål has bought himself a smartwatch, a Fitbit that measures pretty much everything that goes on in his body, including sleep. Now he sends me graphic representations of different nights, readings of his own sleep – a graph with separate colours for the different stages of sleep. After a night out on the town, he has slept seven hours – of which one hour is split between deep and REM sleep. The rest of the night, six hours, was spent in light sleep or awake. After a normal night without alcohol he slept eight hours: one hour of deep sleep, one hour of REM sleep, and the rest either light sleep or wakefulness. Njål seems confused by the graphs. *I don't feel as if the Fitbit is quite working properly*, he says.

It'll be a long time before I buy myself a smartwatch. Monitoring the makeup of my own sleep night after night will do me no good whatsoever. Anything that adds to my self-consciousness ruins my sleep. Besides – can you really trust a gadget fastened to your wrist?

After keeping off it for four months, I'm back on Facebook. I post a new status a couple of times a month; normally I just try to be funny. Once in a while, I'll write about something that upsets me (and instantly regret it). I like other people's posts and check whether I've had any likes myself; at first, I used to laugh at this system, but now it's become the reality we must comply with. I read about other authors showing off their achievements – good reviews, foreign sales and so on – exactly the way I show off my own. Using social media isn't something I've missed, but more like an instinct to be suppressed. Why is it so strong, this urge to check what others are doing, what others are saying, what others are thinking? What fundamental instincts require me to keep myself updated about everything at all times and to keep others updated about me? Why, when I am at my daughter's dance class, do I feel compelled to learn that a person I went to school with thirty-five years ago has bought a new light fixture for his kitchen? It makes me neither happy nor contented – quite the contrary. I can't help comparing my own life with the sum of everybody else's, and generally feel nothing but envy or despair at my inability to achieve what others can. To be on Facebook is to be alone in the face of everything, and the insomnia amplifies it all. I become a lonely, power-less insomniac in an ocean of well-rested success stories. I can't talk about my sleep troubles on Facebook either, because the language doesn't exist there. Only when I have overcome my difficulties or somehow converted my defeat into victory (by writing a book about it, say) can sleeplessness be communicated.

Cutting out Facebook was the first step I took when I realised I had to do something about my sleep problems, but I had no good explanation for why it felt necessary – or no medical or psychological explanation at any rate. I simply understood that I had to get out of there. First of all I had to clear up my thoughts; if I was going to sleep better, I needed less noise in my life. Secondly, I had to force some commitment from my thoughts. I had to get back to long thoughts, instead of hopping from one to the next. This doesn't just apply to social media, but to internet use as a whole. Sleeplessness and internet surfing create a vicious circle. The less I have slept the more difficult it becomes to immerse myself in anything at all – writing, a book, an album, a longish train of reasoning. My brain wants whatever will give it quick and easy gains, without committing itself. Facebook, with its stream of commonplaces and absurdities, seems tailor-made for the sleepless brain. It demands no commitment and costs nothing. The same goes for the other platforms. When I haven't slept, this light material is the only thing I seek out. A long report on the election in Pakistan? No thanks. I'd rather click on this link about why mince is better than hamburger meat.

In an effort to limit my mobile use, I've installed an app that shows me how much time I spend on my phone. It's up around two hours a day, sometimes over three. I'm ashamed of myself; I don't want to be a smartphone addict, but as long as I'm not sleeping, I can't leave it alone. That's another vicious circle. And then there are the different PC screens, at home and at work, and all the TV I watch. Every evening as night approaches, I go through the same routine. I switch off the lamp on the shelf above the sofa to avoid staring straight into a light source in the final hours before night – only to continue staring at the TV screen.

In recent years, I've started taking my mobile or an iPad to bed once in a while to watch a film but usually to listen to a podcast. Just lying there, without any kind of stimulus as I did for the first thirty years of my life, is no longer an option.

When I was a child, I was allowed to stand in front of the bookshelf in the living room for two minutes before bedtime choosing the evening's reading matter. It was a two-and-a-half metre floor-to-ceiling bookshelf – no more than three to four hundred books, but for me the choice was infinite. Some evenings I couldn't decide before Mum called me to bed and then I had to grab a book at random. That meant I risked ending up with a seven-hundred-page slave saga or an erotic contemporary novel. Okay, so my parents could have kept more of an eye on what I took to bed with me as a nine-year-old, but that was still better than what I'm exposed to nowadays: everything. Everything ever published in the way of text and image and sound is within my grasp, just a few clicks away as I lie there in bed. The quantity seems to double daily while the number of hours in the day remains constant.

A US survey of 1,500 adults showed that 90 per cent regularly used portable electronic devices in the last hour before bedtime.[57] But technology and our habits aren't the only things that have changed; the light radiating from all these new screens is also new.

LED light is the modern, much more efficient and durable light that is now used in almost all electronic light sources, including all the brightly lit screens we stare at. LED is short for light-emitting diode, and its invention earned three Japanese scientists the Nobel Prize in Physics in 2014. LED light is extremely energy efficient and has a long life span – which is good news when it comes to reducing energy consumption but bad news for human sleeping habits. The light that strikes our eye affects the circadian clock in our brain and its control of melatonin, which triggers the process of falling asleep. Only when light vanishes does the brain understand that the day is over and it is time for bed.

All artificial light is a threat to the natural circadian rhythm. But why is the new LED light worse than the 'old' light of incandescent bulbs?

The spectrum of light visible to us humans runs from cool blue and purple, which are the short wavelengths, to warm yellow and red, the longer wavelengths. Sunlight contains the entire spectrum. LED light contains most of the short wavelengths and it is this short-wavelength light the receptors in our eyes are most sensitive to when the signal about night and day is transmitted to our brain. This sensitivity is something we inherited from our pre-human forebears, which lived in water and developed their sense of sight there. Water filtered out the longer wavelengths, which is why we see water as blue; and that is also why aquatic species and their descendants – in other words, all of us – are more sensitive to blue light.[58]

Fortunately, there are now easy ways to limit our exposure to blue light. According to Walker, blue light does twice as much damage to our circadian rhythm, melatonin secretions and nightly sleep as the warmer, yellower light of a normal incandescent bulb – even though both emit equally high luminosity. A study that monitored healthy adults' sleep after reading a paper book as opposed to a book on an iPad showed how much poorer the participants' sleep quality became when they had stared at a screen before going to bed: melatonin release occurred three hours later and melatonin secretion did not peak before midnight, as it is meant to, but early the following morning.[59] The participants took longer to fall asleep, lost significant amounts of REM sleep, and felt more exhausted and sleepier the following day.

II

My children aren't as corrupted by blue light as I am. They watch TV for an hour or two before going to bed but no more than that. In bed, I read them a book and we sing a song. When they quieten down and fall asleep,

I become sleepy myself as I sit there waiting. Instead of giving in to it, lying down beside them and sleeping, I keep myself awake by surfing on my mobile.

Why don't I lie down and sleep when I feel as if I can? Because I know that if I go to sleep at the same time as the kids, at around eight o'clock, I'll wake up at roughly midnight and be unable to get back to sleep again until dawn. The same thing happens to Line whenever she falls asleep as she's putting the kids to bed. If I sleep at around eight o'clock, that will break the rhythm I'm working so hard to sustain: getting up with the family at 6.30 a.m., getting to work by eight o'clock, coming home at four o'clock, eating dinner and spending time with the family, and then spending the evening with Line or meeting friends before going to bed, conscience clear, at eleven o'clock.

Nowadays, only an eccentric would go to bed at eight o'clock and then spend half the night wandering around, but in previous times it was actually the norm.

In 2001, American history professor Roger Ekirch showed that today's sleeping patterns, involving eight hours of continuous sleep every night, are an innovation.[60] [61] The way Ekirch discovered the old sleeping pattern shared by a large proportion of the world's population also bears witness to the difficulty of acquiring historical information about sleep. All archaeological and historical research is based on the previous activity of *waking* people. How we humans worked, how we ate, how we hunted, which gods we worshipped, how we buried our dead: proof of these exists in everything from small tools that have lain buried in the earth to the vast footprint left by our civilisation. Cities and countries have come into being during humanity's quest to satisfy all its various needs – with the exception of one. When we sleep, we leave no traces for the future. The fact that human sleeping patterns from a few hundred years ago were not discovered until 2001 shows just how inaccessible the history of sleep is.

It all started when Ekirch was working on his original project – writing about night in pre-industrial times. He found incomprehensible references to sleep in sources that included Chaucer's *Canterbury Tales*. The book was written in the late 1300s and in one of the tales, a character is said to rise from 'his first sleep', then later goes back to bed. In the *Odyssey*, Homer also writes about a first sleep. There is a gap of two thousand years between the two works, but both texts show that humans – at least within this period – had two rounds of sleep in the course of the night. They went to bed a short while after sunset and slept for around four hours. Then, at around one in the morning, they woke up again. For a brief time in the middle of the night, people would get up and do what they could in the dark. They had the energy and opportunity to have sex, or they could pray, read, urinate and so on.

Before, it was easier to maintain the rhythm of the light: the sun rose, it became light. When the sun vanished, it became dark, really dark; there wasn't a single light source. Unless there was moonlight, it was impossible to see more than a metre in front of your face. The only thing to do was go to bed and wait for it to become light again, hopefully in a place where you were safe from predators with good night vision.

The planet's orbit was the sole factor determining humanity's supply of light. Circadian rhythm ensured that nobody was in any doubt about what time of day it was. The signals sent to the nucleus suprachiasmaticus were unmistakable: now it is night and time to sleep.

Melatonin was sent out in the brain and sleep came to all.

Let there be light! God's first words, according to the Bible. Since those days, humanity has taken over that job for itself. Humans are visual creatures – more than a third of our brain is dedicated to processing visual information. We orientate ourselves according to what we can see rather than what we can feel, taste or hear. That appears to be why we slowly but surely secured control over the dark part of the day. *So, our species is supposed to spend half its time unable to see, is it? We're not standing for that!*

In a cave in South Africa, archaeologists have found remnants of million-year-old ashes, left by what they assume to be a fire.[62] However, it is unlikely that the light from this fire will have affected our forebears' sleeping habits: beyond the glow of the flames, the world remained dark and unknown. Long after that came wax candles, followed by oil lamps, innovations that altered humans' opportunities to be up after darkness fell – although these light sources didn't exactly set the world ablaze. The first public lamp was hung at the Grand Chatelet in Paris in 1318. Some 560 years later, on 22nd October 1879, Edison managed to make a carbon filament light up for 13.5 hours. Electric light had arrived. The night was the last great continent left for humanity to conquer and explore. At last darkness was forced to give way – and sleep along with it.

An American experiment, carried out at roughly the same time as Ekirch made his discoveries, found traces of this ancient sleeping pattern in modern humans.[63] Researchers removed all artificial light sources from a group of people, leaving them exposed only to daylight. They spent fourteen hours a day in darkness. For the first few weeks they slept as usual, the way all modern humans do, with continuous nightly sleep. But then the pattern shifted: they started to wake after midnight and didn't go back to sleep for a good hour. Blood tests showed that the subjects' stress levels were at their lowest during this hour between the first and second sleep. They lapsed into the sleeping pattern our forebears followed several hundred years ago. In the few inhabited places on Earth that are not yet illuminated, there are still people who sleep in two shifts.[64]

III

Hi insomniacs!

This is how I start a post on Reddit. I write that I want to make contact with young people who have sleep difficulties. I publish it and wait a few days but receive no replies. Either nobody wants to talk to me about this topic or I've got too old to work out where and how to make contact with young people.

I was born in the age of TV, radio and incandescent bulbs. In the seventies, my parents generally sat up watching TV for several hours after sunset. Then maybe they'd take a book or a magazine to bed. They slept continuous sleep and usually had a lie-in the next morning if it was a day off, until long after the sun had risen. This is the pattern I continued in my own adult life with just a few, if marked, changes in the TV on offer during the eighties and nineties. Only when I was in my mid-thirties did the smartphone and Facebook arrive.

But what about the people who don't know a world any different from the one we live in today? What relationship do they have to the new technology and how does its use affect their sleep? *It's especially serious among young adults and youths in sixth form,* sleep scientist Børge Sivertsen told me when he spoke about the incidence of insomnia in the Norwegian population. If that's true, what's the reason?

Liv, my sleep-yoga buddy, has worked in a sixth-form college for more than ten years and says she is seeing a scary development in young people's sleeping habits. Technological advances are partly to blame, she thinks.

'Ten years ago, we saw clear signs among certain boys at school who were addicted to gaming. They'd sit up playing at night, come to school late and of course it affected their schoolwork, and in the end a lot of them dropped out,' Liv says after one of our yoga sessions, adding: 'But things have got worse for more people since smartphones arrived.'

Liv tells me about going on a field trip to a tourist cabin with one class. All the mobile phones were confiscated for the duration of the trip, which is normal practice.

'Some of the kids were totally frantic at the idea of going to bed without their mobile phones. They had no idea what they were going to do to get to sleep.'

'Sounds like me,' I say.

'When I talk to them about their poor sleeping habits, a lot of them say they've been struggling with sleep for years. And when I suggest that they should go to bed without their phones, they say that's no good because then what are they supposed to do in the four hours they'll spend lying awake? It's like talking to an alcoholic. The thing that is destroying them is the one thing they think can help them. I see so many tired kids who arrive late, sit there freezing in the classrooms and fall asleep during lessons.'

Liv sighs. 'It's as if we live in a society where nobody values sleep anymore.'

One afternoon two weeks later I get a message from a Reddit administrator; they accidentally deleted my post to sleepless young people and have only just found out. If I want, they write, I can post the message again.

I give it another try. If there are any sleepless people out there who want to talk to me, get in touch, I write. Then I send a mail to the administrator to make sure they won't delete it again. Just as I'm shutting my laptop, I get a mail from an unknown address.

I saw your post on Reddit. I've been struggling with sleep to varying degrees all my life and use medicine to get to sleep.

Somebody has answered after just two minutes! Eagerly, I start to formulate a reply: I can't think how to tackle this – I just want to send the person a response. But before I can complete it, a new mail comes in.

I'm a 19-year-old boy and for as long as I can remember I've had real trouble sleeping.

And another:

I'm a 22-year-old man with a lot of sleep problems. If you want to talk to me, just get in touch.

As I read the third e-mail yet another one ticks in, this one from a young musician who has developed such bad sleeping habits on tour that he can't get to sleep when he comes home. And yet another one after that, from a young boy who hasn't slept normally since he was little.

Over the next few hours, e-mails pour in from sleepless people across the country, most of them in their early or mid-twenties, some younger. Mostly young men. So many young people who aren't sleeping! Over the days that follow the e-mails continue to pour in, and with them my panic rises. I asked for insomniacs and I got insomniacs.

But what do I do now?

In some cases, it's difficult to interpret the severity: when they say they're struggling with sleep, do they just have a bad night now and then, the way all humans do? In other cases, there's no room for doubt: the senders tell me about prolonged, severe sleep problems, about the medicines they take and all the other solutions they have tried. I don't want to interview people I later realise aren't suffering from insomnia. And yet I don't want to brush aside anybody who does have severe sleep disorders. Another thing I mustn't forget when I talk to young people complaining about their sleep is that many of them may have a delayed sleep phase – in other words, their youth means they are genetically predisposed to go to bed and get up later than school and society require them to. This isn't the same as insomnia, despite the resemblance: terrible sleeping habits, poor sleep, minimal surplus energy in their everyday life.

To find out more about each individual, I respond to all of them with the same questions: *Is your sleep difficulty so severe that it affects your days? Can you briefly describe how you sleep?* Some I never hear from again. Most of the e-mails arrived in the middle of the night or late in the evening. Maybe in some desperate sleepless moment the senders simply wanted to send out a cry for help. Maybe when my response reaches them they have had a good night's sleep and no longer see any point in speaking to somebody about insomnia. Those who reply do so comprehensively, telling me in detail how long they lie awake, how many times they wake up in the night, what medicines they take, all the other options they have tried, how long they have struggled with sleep. As certain cases crystallise into the people I should talk to, I can't repress my delight: the sleep scientist was right!

'My sleep problems started some time in Year Six or Seven. I had a lot of bad habits, like too much screen time before bed. A lot of gaming in the evenings, TV, mobile, those sorts of distractions. Then I'd lie awake longer and longer into the night before getting to sleep. And whenever I got bored, I'd get out the Playstation or my mobile.'

Markus is twenty-one and it's a couple of years since he left sixth-form college. He can't get to sleep until late at night and often ends up lying awake until daybreak. Markus is one of many young people whose sleeping habits have been ruined by too much screen time and stimulation. What started in primary school only became worse in sixth form. After sleepless nights it was difficult to get up in the mornings and that started to take a toll on his school attendance and marks.

He's the first one I've managed to contact by phone. You have to be flexible if you want to make arrangements with young people outside the margins of normal professional and family life who are also struggling to sleep at normal times. It's late in the evening when I finally get to talk to him. He answers my questions politely.

'Almost every day I arrived late. If I got there on time it was because I hadn't slept. And then I might just as well not have turned up. If I've slept too little, I'm heavy-headed. It affects my mood, my concentration –

everything, really. I often didn't get to school before eleven o'clock. Luckily my teachers turned a blind eye to my absence. I tried various sleep aids, including melatonin, but they had almost no effect. In my last year, my tactic was to go home and sleep straight after school, wake up at one in the morning and stay awake until school started and then throughout the rest of the day, all to avoid failing my course because of poor attendance.'

'Were you the only one struggling with sleep?'

'No, there were a few of us in my class.'

Nowadays Markus works in the afternoon, as a sales manager at a call centre, and feels that he gets the sleep he needs. But not without medication.

'Before I used to take Vallergan, which made me sleep but had unbelievable side effects. It felt as if I'd been boozing for ten days. Now I take Truxal. It makes me tired and it suppresses the racing thoughts too.'

'Do you brood a lot?'

'Yes, I find myself trapped in lots of different trains of thought and then I just lie there, unable to sleep. I'm easily distracted and impatient. If I'm not tired, I quickly take out my mobile or a book.'

'Do you have a plan?' I ask. 'I mean, with the pills. Do you and your doctor have a plan?'

What I'm really wondering is this: *You're at the start of your life and these sleep difficulties may get in the way of studies, work and a normal social life. What has your doctor thought of doing about these difficulties apart from giving you pills that only help you one night at a time?*

'I'm not always going to need the pills. But for now things are working as well as they can. I don't think I'd consider stopping them any time soon. I know the pills are a short-term solution. I'll be starting university and that takes discipline. So I'm going to have to force myself to get out of bed. At sixth-form college I didn't have that discipline. I'm a bit more grown-up now. Maybe I'll manage to sort out my circadian rhythm,' Markus says.

A few days later, I make Skype contact with Stian, the second sleepless young man I speak to.

'I sleep three or four hours before waking up in the middle of the night and then I can't get back to sleep,' he tells me. 'I try but it just doesn't work. So I flip open my laptop and sit there with it for a few hours before going to school. Then there's the problem of getting through the day. I struggle to concentrate even in the morning. If anything distracts me, I zone out. Then I go home and sleep until I feel rested, anything from one to three hours. I have to sleep if I'm going to get out and meet other people and feel as if I have a life. But I don't always manage to sleep in the afternoons either. I end up lying awake and feeling the pressure to get some sleep. Electronic devices have a big impact on my sleep,' he tells me. 'The feeling that we have to be available twenty-four hours a day, I think it affects my sleep – and a lot of other people's too.'

Stian got hooked on World of Warcraft when he was twelve. And that altered his sleeping habits: he started to go to bed late and slept badly throughout secondary school. Now he's studying to be a social worker in Bodø and his sleep difficulties have become much worse. He's on Seroquel, which is prescribed as a sedative. Previously he has taken Vallergan. Stian tells me he is going through a long depression, without offering further details. In 2018 he was hospitalised on a ward for mild mental disorders. Over his seven-week stay he slept well. Here, too, technology – or rather its absence – played an important role.

'The ward had problems with its Wi Fi network and I

couldn't get online in the evenings. So I started reading books or playing board games or talking to the other people there. By the end of my stay and when I came out again, I was falling asleep after half an hour and sleeping eight or nine hours every night. So, logging off really helped. I heard recently that the Wi Fi is back up on the ward. And now everybody sits in their rooms surfing.'

'If you see obvious improvements in your sleep from logging off,' I say, 'why do you log back on again?'

'I don't know. It's a difficult habit to break. I did some supervised training at a secondary school a year back and I noticed there how scary it is with social media. They really go the extra mile to keep users hooked, especially young people who are easy to manipulate. The pupils there used to send each other pointless pictures on Snapchat just to keep their streaks going. All the relationships between the young people were linked to the telephone. They would call each other at night and most of them expected everybody to be available,' Stian says, adding: 'Sleep deprivation is a widespread problem for lots and lots of secondary school pupils. And just like me they keep their phones beside their bed at night to check if anybody has tried to get in touch with them or if anything important has happened. It's a kind of addiction. I've installed software to dim the screen so that I won't sit staring at blue light before I'm supposed to be going to sleep.'

Towards the end of our conversation, I can no longer restrain myself.

'I have a tip for you,' I say. 'There's a treatment method for people like us, and sleep scientists agree that it's the best one.'

'Oh?' says Stian.

'I'm going to try it myself next week,' I say.

160

NOVEMBER

The Breakfast Club

I

'Sleep people!'

Some people get up, while others remain seated. All of us in the small, wet-floored, sniffling waiting room of Lovisenberg Diakonale Hospital are strangers to each other. It's the penultimate day in October and the snow has made its first incursion, although the five centimetres that settled over Oslo during the night are already being washed away by rain. I have spent the wait trying to work out who is here for sleep difficulties and who is here for other reasons. It's difficult to spot social markers or demographic indicators of any kind; everybody is sitting there in dark winter jackets, mobile phones glued to their faces. Every time I'm certain I've identified another insomniac, he or she is called in by other therapists.

But now at last it is our turn.

'Everybody who's going to the Sleep School, follow me!'

Only now that we are called in and stand up do I see who's who. The therapist doesn't wait for us: no sooner has he stuck his head in and called out than he's gone again, and we do our best to keep up. The place so smacks of local government it could be used as a historical film set: stark lighting from the low ceiling and shining linoleum floors – the sexiest thing in here is the rust-red brick walls. And of course, those silver-grey signs with glued-on black letters that somebody hung up, all over Norway, sometime in the seventies. We go along one corridor, then another, and after that we pass through what must be the staff canteen, then out into a new corridor and up a narrow staircase. Here we come to a halt in a long column, because there's some fuss about the meeting room, but then everything turns out to be fine after all. We drift into a little room, just as dismal and cramped as all the rest of the building. A big round skylight could have helped lift the mood but right now, all it offers is a dark-grey late autumn afternoon sky. What's more, there's a grille in front of the glass.

Have there been many escape attempts from here?

We organise the chairs and tables, all rickety, arranging ourselves in a square so that we all sit facing one another. There is a solidarity and hopefulness to the activity. We don't know each other; know nothing about one another except that we are all here to sleep better.

We settle. Nervous smiles and glances. At last I can look around me. It's fascinating, I notice, to observe a group of people and know that *everybody here sleeps badly*. If I hadn't known that the purpose of this gathering was to achieve better sleep, I never would have guessed it. But what did I expect? Something like the cast of an Ingmar Bergman film, maybe? Gaunt, faded women and highly educated men with receding hairlines and a penchant for making life difficult for themselves.

Instead, the people I see are perfectly ordinary. Not individually, but as a group, they form an utterly normal gathering of Norwegians; we could just as easily be sitting on the Underground in central Oslo on a Thursday morning. Beside me sits a giant of a man in a plumber's uniform with tattooed hands and forearms. He'd never have made it through the auditions for a Bergman film, but here he sits. On my other side is a middle-aged woman who looks as if she might run a smallholding. Then comes an elderly man, a woman from an immigrant background, a couple of representatives of the more down-at-heel segment of the population, both knees and voices cracking. Only one person here appears to share my demographic traits: a man of my own age who's already sitting there asleep.

Seven women and five men. Twelve in all.

The sleep people.

The two therapists introduce themselves cautiously, almost hesitantly. Are they afraid we might fall apart at any moment? Or is it because they're doing this for the first time? But no, they have worked at the Sleep School for the past two or three years, they tell us. The Sleep School and this treatment have existed for ten years.

Ten years! If only I could have sat here ten years ago. I still don't know whether this will help but I have a feeling that I've never been closer.

This is the method the American Medical Association has concluded should be the primary treatment option for all insomnia patients, the one mentioned by all three sleep scientists I have spoken to and what sleep scientist Børge Sivertsen refers to as the *gold standard*. Scientists call it cognitive behavioural therapy for insomnia (CBTi). In 2018, the impressively named *National Recommendation for the Study and Treatment of Insomnia* concluded that this treatment 'is recommended as the first choice for chronic insomnia in adults over eighteen.' It is well documented that eight out of ten patients who follow this method experience significant improvement in their sleep, and the effects are lasting. A Norwegian study also shows that the treatment works better than sleep medicine.[65]

So, what does this gold standard entail?

The treatment may be administered individually, in the form of group therapy or even as self-help, and one fundamental idea is that it can be adapted to each individual case. Traditionally, it consists of a selection of five different elements: sleep hygiene, stimulus control, sleep restriction, cognitive techniques and relaxation techniques.

Everybody around the table has attended a personal consultation with one of the therapists. A brief chat – I don't think I sat there longer than fifteen minutes. I offered my history, in what has become an almost routine presentation for me over the past eight months: my sleep difficulties – what, how and when, although not so much why. When I mentioned my good and bad patches, the way I could be on a high one week and plunge into the depths the next, and how my sleeping patterns preceded or followed these peaks and troughs, the therapist shrugged.

'It could be something called cyclothymia,' he said before continuing with his questions.

Only when I came for my first consultation did I discover that the Sleep School was just a couple of minutes' walk from my own home. I didn't know whether to laugh or cry. I have scoured the city in search of a cure for sleeplessness and the most obvious option is right across the street.

The setting reminds me of the kind of group therapy I've seen on TV: twelve different people with pretty much the same ailment, each speaking in turn. Tears, intimate and intense tales of our messed-up lives.

Suddenly I get nervous. Do I have anything to tell? Do I have *a story*? There's a swish of rainproof jackets. One person sniffs. Another coughs. One of the psychologists gets up and adjusts the position of a whiteboard in a corner of the cramped meeting room.

Circadian rhythm control, he writes, then looks at us.

'This involves getting up at the same time every morning, weekdays and weekends. You can choose this time yourselves. Whatever suits you best. But once you've chosen it, you have to stick to it, every day.'

A new term: *Stimulus control*.

'You need to teach your brain to associate your bedroom and your bed with sleep and nothing but sleep, so you can only lie awake in your bed for twenty minutes. If you haven't fallen asleep in that time, you must get up and leave the bedroom.'

Finally, he writes *Sleep deprivation*.

'The idea is that each night, you will lie in bed no longer than the amount of time you currently sleep. If you sleep an average of six hours a night, you mustn't lie in bed for more than six hours. But nobody must lie there for fewer than five-and-a-half hours. That's a minimum. Less than that is indefensible. You must find a length of time that suits you and stick to it every night, week after week. Then we'll gradually increase that length of time.'

The other therapist takes over.

'For example,' he says, 'if you sleep an average of six hours and have to get up at seven o'clock to get to work on time, you'll need to stay awake until one in the morning. *You are not allowed to go to bed before that*. What's more, if you wake up at four o'clock and can't get back to sleep, you must get out of bed after lying awake for twenty minutes. Then you must wait until you feel tired enough before going back to bed. You must get up at seven o'clock and you must stay up until one o'clock the following morning, no matter what. The idea is to create sleep pressure that overrides all the other things that make you lie awake. Think of it as being hit over the head with a hammer to make you sleep. You'll get very tired, so we tend to advise patients not to make any big decisions in the six-week duration of the treatment. It may also be a good idea to tell your nearest and dearest that you'll be behaving strangely over the coming weeks, okay?'

The therapists sit down. Silence falls and in the quiet, nervousness seems to spread through the room until one of them starts speaking again.

'Let's go around the table.'

Here come the tears, I think. Now we'll tell each other about ourselves and how dreadfully we sleep.

But no, the only thing we're supposed to share is the time we've decided to get up and when we can go to bed.

'I have to be at work by nine o'clock,' says the first person, a young woman. 'So I have to get up at eight.'

'And how many hours do you usually sleep a night?' asks one of the therapists.

'Three or four.'

'Then you can lie in bed for five-and-a-half hours, which means that you can go to bed at...'

'2.30 a.m.?' the woman says, laughing nervously as the reality of the treatment dawns on her, on all of us.

Soon it's my turn. It isn't new to me, this idea that getting up at the same time every day is good for your circadian rhythm and, by extension, your sleep. It's one of the tips that is always listed in newspaper articles about how to sleep better, and one of the few that is simple and easy to understand. I opt for 6.30 a.m., which is the time I've been getting up lately anyway, mostly because of the two-year-old. 6.30 a.m., that means I have to stay up until one o'clock. On average I sleep fewer than five-and-a-half hours so that will be my length of time. It doesn't sound all that difficult, I think. I don't sleep any more than that anyway. The challenge will be dropping my daytime naps, those minutes of shuteye I'm in the habit of taking when the sleep deprivation gets too much.

After everybody has said their time out loud, it goes quiet again. The therapists sit there with encouraging little smiles on their lips, nothing more. I realise the appointment is over and look at the clock. We haven't been here more than forty minutes. So there won't be a round of whinging after all; it basically seems as if the two therapists are trying to avoid it. It looks as though that isn't part of the treatment. Not yet, at any rate. Just as well, I think as I let my gaze slide over the other eleven, that way I get out of hearing about the problems of strangers. But I sense that I'm a bit disappointed too. I had, I now realise, resigned myself to the idea that we would compare war wounds:

A good night is maybe three hours' sleep.
Ha! I don't get more than a couple of hours a night.
Lucky bastards, I don't sleep more than an hour, max!

We're handed a form and told to fill in the time we go to bed, when we get up, how many times we wake up in the night and, finally, what percentage of the time we have slept. Everybody picks up their papers and then we drift out of the little meeting room, each going our separate ways. None of us have exchanged a word, we haven't introduced ourselves, we have hardly looked at each other, we sleep people.

II

The first night. The family is sleeping and it's ten o'clock. I have to stay awake for another three hours. This isn't an unfamiliar situation for me – the others going to bed, me staying up. But there's one important difference: tonight going to bed before one o'clock is not *allowed*. This actually gives me a certain control. Sleepiness starts to waft over me at around eleven o'clock, both earlier and heavier than normal. I sit in front of the TV, eyes drooping. I have to get up, go out into the kitchen and do some clearing up to avoid falling asleep on the sofa.

If I tell my own brain to sleep, I liven up. If I refuse to let it sleep, as now, I can barely keep my eyes open. In a way, it's the opposite of Daniel Wegner's experiment with the Walkman in the eighties. Instead of being instructed to fall asleep as quickly as possible, my homework is to stay awake – yes, to sleep as little as possible. Fit to drop, I wander around the flat until ten to one. Then I brush my teeth. The final goal is, of course, to sleep well in my own bed; but there, the danger of being woken by the kids during the night is far too great. And the time I am allowed to sleep has suddenly been restricted. I go to bed on the sofa.

One step at a time.

31st October: Go to bed at 1 a.m. get up 6.30 a.m. Slept at 1.10 a.m. Woke up twice for fifteen minutes. Sleep efficiency: 87 per cent.

The next morning I fill in the form, which isn't like a journal, because there's no room for the subjective; it's all times and numbers. Since I lay on the sofa for five-and-a-half hours and was awake for forty minutes, my sleep efficiency is 87 per cent. Part of the treatment is to be as objective as possible. Don't think, don't try, don't complicate matters, just follow the rules and write down the numbers. But of course, I can't escape the subjective: I feel rested. Those almost five hours of sleep have given me the energy boost that will take me through the day and into the night. It's Halloween and I'm painting my face before going out with my daughter in search of sweets. During the evening, I forget the system; only when I start yawning at around eleven o'clock, do I remember.

Ah, the treatment! I can't go to bed until one o'clock.

I put on a film and lie down on the sofa. Fixed frameworks. Control. Extra time to sit up late *and* better sleep when I eventually go to bed. Six weeks of this – of course I'll manage. And then I'll be cured! At one o'clock, I settle for the night. After ten minutes the boy calls out. I go into his room and he calms down quickly. Then I go back to bed and go to sleep, but an hour later he's awake again.

1st November: Go to bed at 1 a.m. Sleep at 1.10 a.m. Woken up for thirty minutes. Wake up at 4 a.m. and can't sleep again. Sleep efficiency: ?

I can't do this. Since I'm not allowed to lie awake in bed for more than twenty minutes, I'm already up by 4.30 a.m. I'm not going to get any more sleep tonight – neither the good, deep sleep nor the light, useless dozing. Right now, I'd happily have accepted anything at all; I'm queasy and dizzy. My head is hot and my throat sore, as if a cold is just lying there waiting for another sleepless night. I hold it together through the morning routines, help dress the kids and drop them off, get to the office and work as normal for an hour before falling apart. Everything stops dead. The afternoon is like a desert: no landmarks, just hour after hour of wandering: work, pick-up at the kindergarten, dinner, washing up, supper, bedtime. A brain incapable of sorting and so bereft of sleep that it cannot establish a distance between itself and its surroundings: my entire being is implicated in even the tiniest tasks. I take teaspoons out of the dishwasher and put them in the cutlery drawer. I can barely hold out but I have to wait! Keep it up until I make it to one o'clock, when I can shut my eyes.

2nd Nov.: Go to bed at 1 a.m., sleep at 1.10 a.m. Woke up twice, for fifteen and thirty minutes. Sleep efficiency: ?

3rd Nov.: Go to bed at 1 a.m., sleep at 1.15 a.m. Woke up twice for thirty and sixty minutes. Sleep efficiency: ?

The amount of time I can spend in bed is shorter than I am used to, and as I lie there it feels as if I am sleeping more poorly than normal. On paper it looks as though I have slept, but it's light sleep, wretched sleep. And then there's the business of the boy at night, which the people who developed the treatment couldn't possibly have foreseen. I can go to bed at one o'clock but my son may still wake around that time and disturb me. He has been waking up like this for several months, but only now do I realise how disruptive it is for the treatment.

The queasiness and headache dog me throughout the day. I can't write, can't work – I can barely manage to be there for the family. After dropping the boy off on Friday morning, I realise that I've walked several hundred metres still wearing the protective plastic covers from the kindergarten over the top of my shoes. Saturday is the worst – almost no sleep at night and we're supposed to spend the entire day together. I withdraw; all I want to do is sink into my mobile and surf inanities. The worst of it is the doubt and despondency. I'm so frazzled that every aspect of my life looks like a mistake. All roads lead straight into the depths. Why am I seeking success as a writer? Why do I keep making music after all these years? Why do I, in all my mediocrity, try to do anything at all?

At the same time, I'm capable of seeing myself from the outside and holding onto the knowledge that sleep is what is doing this to me – or lack of sleep. An hour's snooze and the meaning will seep back into my life again. Now it's just a matter of holding out until Tuesday and the next meeting with the therapists and the group.

Ah, the tales I shall tell them.

4th Nov.: Go to bed at 1 a.m. Sleep at 1.10 a.m. Wake up at 6 a.m. Sleep efficiency: 87.

One night of decent sleep and everything is reversed again. We clear the garden and then I take the children to the swimming pool. I'm strong, I'm contented and I'm present. I start to make plans again. Books I'll write, songs I'll record; we'll redecorate the dining room, we'll go on a trip. Evening comes and as the others start to get tired, I decide to make a list of everything that needs to be done to the flat. A handful of hours of continuous deep sleep is all I need. I'm so full of life that when night comes, I don't get sleepy; although I go to bed at one o'clock, I lie there wide awake. I don't want to rest now, I just want to carry on. I get up again and go to bed again and get up again. God almighty. I'm so pathetic. I have no control, can't function as a human being. All it takes is a few hours' shuteye and I'm so wound up I can't sleep for the next two nights. How can I be so easily hurled down into the depths and then, just as swiftly, hauled up to the heights of ecstasy?

Will I never be in balance?

What is wrong with me?

One night while I'm lying on the sofa in front of the TV waiting for one o'clock to arrive, I watch a programme starring a British illusionist. He gives four people with different phobias sugar pills and tricks them into believing that it's real medicine designed to cure fear. After a few weeks, three of the four have overcome their phobias. The man who is scared witless of social contact and confrontation stops a bar fight; the man who is scared of heights and bridges is capable of standing on the parapet of a bridge fifty metres above the water. Then the illusionist tells the participants the truth: the medicine was fake. You found these new paths in your mind all by yourselves, he tells them. Their faith in the cure is removed – but they remain cured.

There's something reassuring about coming into the waiting room and seeing the collection of faces from the previous Tuesday again. If I'd walked past any one of them on the street, I wouldn't have reacted. We don't even meet each other's gaze when we're going in and out. But now we gather: one after another, we come into the waiting room and become a community. One of the women looks like an older version of the American actress Ally Sheedy and I think we're like a slightly less photogenic version of *The Breakfast Club* – people who would never have had anything to do with one another in the outside world but all share the same flaw in here.

Two of the women exchange their experiences of the past week, speaking so quietly I can barely hear them:

How did it go?

I've managed to follow the system at least. I slept well but I don't know whether it's the treatment or just a good patch. What about you?

Then we're taken into a room; it's bigger, brighter and more pleasant than last time.

A new room. Is that part of the therapy?

We sit in a horseshoe formation, and only now do we discover that there are just eleven of us this time. Pens and paper are handed out and the therapists go around the table.

'How have you slept?'

Stolen glances as we realise that, for the first time, we'll be allowed to give long and complicated answers to this question. It's what we're here for. But most importantly of all, the therapists particularly want to hear about each person's *sleep efficiency*. If they sleep the moment their head hits the pillow and wake only when the alarm goes off, their sleep efficiency is 100 per cent. If they've lain in bed for six hours but slept only four, the percentage is sixty-six. All of us here know that anybody who has scored an average of more than 80 per cent over the past week may go to bed a quarter of an hour sooner. It means the cure has worked so well that the person has permission to go to bed earlier.

I take out my sleep form and try to sort out the numbers. The first night, I was up at 87 per cent, the second, down to 45 per cent. Very good at first, horribly bad after that. I get no further, not just because my brain is too tired to deal with the figures but also because the figures I've written down are unreliable. Yes, I slept for five-and-a-half hours on the third night, but it was feather-light sleep, useless sleep. And most of my awakenings were caused by the children not my own sleep disorder. The Eastern Front not the Western Front.

The first person to report is a young woman. Her sleeping time was from 00.30 a.m. to six o'clock – she's followed the system despite being dead tired in the evenings, and she has slept through every night, she tells us.

The therapists listen to her, the way I remember my own psychiatrist listening to me: as if they're sitting with a recording that must play to the end; only when the tape stops will they switch out of listening mode and embark hesitantly, almost reluctantly, upon an answer.

'But that's really good,' says the first one.

'Really, really good,' repeats the other one.

The young woman's sleep efficiency is well over 90 per cent and she can start going to bed a quarter of an hour earlier.

The next person has also seen positive effects from the treatment. Her sleep efficiency is over 80 per cent, she can also advance. The third, a middle-aged man, is a bearer of good news, too. We see the joy in his face as he tells us he has seen evident improvements after the first week.

'I haven't slept properly for a year but now...'

He smiles and nods.

So far, everybody around the table has achieved good results in the first week of treatment. My overwhelming feeling is how dispiriting it is not to be among them, I notice. It reminds me of the feeling I get after spending time on Facebook: am I the only one who isn't a success?

And yet I also notice that the others' good results motivate me to go home and persist. If it works for them, surely it must work for me too. I *will* get better!

'It's been up and down,' I say, when my turn comes. 'Mostly down. The first night went well but after that it went pretty badly. I haven't managed to work out a percentage because even though I get to sleep, my sleep is very light and poor. And I haven't managed to sleep in my bed – I'm still sleeping on the sofa. What's more, my two-year-old son has a habit of waking up at around one o'clock, which is when I go to bed and am preparing to fall asleep. He wakes me up again and keeps us all awake, and on top of all that, my sleep treatment feels like a burden I'm imposing on the whole family.'

In the long silence between my report and the therapists' response, I get the sense that I've ruined the mood. It was all going so well, with everyone managing to stick to their numbers and percentages. I'm the first one to whinge.

'But it's great that you're not sleeping!' the therapist says, throwing his arms wide. "Because that's the point.'

I start to understand the thinking behind cognitive therapy: always looking on the bright side. Seeing the positive, steering away from the problems and aiming for the solutions. It's consoling and, to an extent, constructive. But it's also irritatingly transparent, I notice. There's a danger of losing the human aspect, for the response to become mechanical: *You haven't slept for a week? You're incapable of working or spending time with your family? You're starting to get depressed? FANTASTIC!* I nod, realising that there isn't much more I can say. I must either stick to the system and turn up here once a week with my numbers or I must drop out.

After me, as if I mark the watershed, come all the other people around the table who *haven't* slept. And after the introductory success stories, the rest of the group seems disappointed. The huge plumber sounds bitter as he tells us about his week.

"Haven't slept a wink,' he says tersely. 'So I don't know what the people on the other side of the table have been doing.'

'I get stressed out by all the rules,' says one of the women.

'The rigid rules are the whole point,' says one of the therapists. 'The idea is that you'll manage to sleep *despite* the rules.'

Then it's over; we've sat here for barely forty-five minutes before being sent home to our numbers and hours.

Drop the treatment?

Like hell.

I've come this far.

I'm carrying on.

III

Round up the usual suspects, says Captain Renault in the cinema classic, *Casablanca*. That's exactly what I do every time I'm trying to find an explanation for why I sleep so poorly.

I live a life that doesn't add up. This is a thought that often strikes me when I'm juggling my everyday existence: I have two small children I'm trying to give the world's best childhood, a wife I want to make happy, a large circle of family and friends I'm trying to maintain relationships with, a home and a job that sustains my interest. On top of all that I have yet, aged forty-five, to abandon my dream of becoming an acclaimed author, musician *and* author of cartoons. Every single day, my thoughts and actions involve all these aspects of my existence. As the doctor said: sounds like a lot. In addition, there's that pressure all of us are under to be constantly available: for telephone calls, e-mails, status updates, news alerts. Things pour in from all sides. It's a life like anybody else's, but that doesn't improve matters. A medieval man wouldn't have survived a day of it. Samuel Johnson and Benjamin Franklin would have screamed for a less complex daily life and more sleep. Even nineties me would have had problems keeping up today.

Another explanation: insomnia tightened its grip when I stopped studying and started working. I had to get up in the mornings after eight or nine years as a student. In those years, I'd had an extremely irregular circadian rhythm: I played in a band, I drank, I was always one of the last people to leave the after-party and after several days of partying I could sleep for as many days again. Not ideal for a person already susceptible to sleep difficulties. Maybe my lifestyle destroyed all my good sleeping habits; maybe I only noticed the impact of this once I was forced into a 'normal' existence.

Suspect number three: the fear of missing out. Too much freedom isn't good for me but I didn't understand that sixteen years ago. In those days, the world was my oyster. I was going to succeed at everything all at once. I was incapable of saying no. Was it the fear of not opening every door that was the start of my sleep problems?

And then there are my personality traits. Being liked and pleasing other people – whether those close to me or strangers – are things I've always been annoyingly concerned about. Whether it's an exaggerated sense of empathy or just an egotistical desire to be popular I don't know. Maybe both. I feel an almost constant sense of unease about unresolved issues with the people around me.

More explanations: ever since I was a boy, I've found it difficult to keep calm. Once I've hit a high, it can take me hours or even days to come back down. This applies to everything that enthuses or stresses me: being with people, making music, writing or working. I let myself get carried away, nothing can go fast enough and I'm incapable of stopping; it's like an obsession. Sleep is impossible. Rather than just being a result, sleeplessness also serves as a regulator. *Ah, so you can't calm down?* says insomnia. *Well, let's keep you awake for forty-eight hours and see if that helps.*

I have good patches and I have bad patches. I'm way up high and way down low. Before, I used to think that these shifts were always triggered by extreme circumstances in life, but now I'm no longer so sure. Sleep does play a role, that much I know. Am I bipolar? Or, as the psychologist suggested, do I have cyclothymia – a kind of bipolar-lite, according to Wikipedia.

After sixteen years of insomnia, I'm starting to realise that it may not be all that constructive to waste too much time and energy on *why*. *The underlying causes*, as the doctor said, or the answers the psychiatrist sought in my dreams. Too much time has passed. The different factors have all got muddled up. It's no longer possible to pick out a single explanation. It's like a fragment that has embedded itself so deep within the machinery that it's become part of the machine itself. Asking *Why can't I sleep at night* is the same as asking the question *Why am I the way I am*? Maybe it's because I work with storytelling that I've been so obsessed with the thought of cause and origin. But all the other sleepless people who have been through psychotherapy tell me the psychologists also asked them the same questions: there must be something; there must be a *reason* why you don't sleep. Art and psychology both bear within them the same fundamental idea: that everything must have meaning. Everything leads to everything. It's like the famous Chekhov quote: 'If in Act One you have a pistol hanging on the wall, then it must fire in the last act,' only the other way around. If there is a man lying sleepless in the last act, then something must have happened in Act One.

The idea that you are your own past and can never escape it – it's an idea I can no longer be trapped in.

This is not a three-act play.

This is my life.

Your thoughts are free, sang Norwegian singer-songwriter Alf Cranner. But isn't the brain, trapped in its human tower, entirely a hostage to the behaviour of the body it sits atop? If you change your behaviour, your thoughts will follow. Forget cause. Don't think too much about the problems. Or rather, don't think about them at all. Insomnia originates in the mental, on the inside, so the solution must come from the outside. Break down the old pattern and the rest will follow. Don't try because trying springs from an ideal, and the ideal exists only in thoughts. Just do it. Or to turn around the mantra of the old Funkadelic song:

Free your ass, and your mind will follow.

III

It's mid-November, approaching the darkest part of the year. The kids are restless at night – I'm woken before I've fallen asleep, or just lie there awake, waiting for somebody to cry out. The few hours the treatment allows me to sleep must be spent on them. There's so much activity at night that Line and I take turns. Several days, weeks without proper sleep; my back's aching, I'm stiff and sore. One of the short cuts out of our building involves getting over a low fence between the garden and the street. If I've slept well, I leap over it with no difficulty. Now I'm like an old timer: everything goes slowly, everything costs effort and I generally fall over. And even the simple act of falling is something I'm incapable of without enough sleep: it's as if my body has no shock absorbers – the impact with the ground goes straight through me. I get up and carry on walking to the Sleep School. After three weeks, there are only nine of us left around the table. Since the start, three of us have fallen by the wayside. We go around the table. One person after another complains about how difficult the system is, how tired they are, how disappointed they are that the improvement is not happening faster. But when the therapists ask how high their sleep efficiency is, all of them have over eighty-five! Well then; that'll be a quarter of an hour earlier to bed for you, they say. Oh right, answer the people who are sleeping so much better. That's true.

Don't they realise how lucky they are? Don't they see that the system is working? Are they incapable of taking pleasure in the reward they receive for their efforts? High sleep efficiency – almost at the same level as a normal person – and a quarter of an hour earlier to bed every week.

How *dare* they complain?

Now it's the middle-aged man's turn – the one who was moved to tears the first week when he discovered that the treatment helped. This time he tells us about a bad week. He slept well the first four nights, he says, but then his grandchildren came to stay for three nights.

'It was all just a mess,' he tells us, shaking his head.

That's when it dawns on me. This can't go on. It doesn't help that I have *decided* to sleep well between 1 a.m. and 6.30 a.m. It doesn't help that I believe the treatment will work, that I am more motivated than ever before. I sit up until one o'clock every night but when I go to bed, I am constantly disturbed, and when I get up at 6.30 a.m., I can't even manage to fill in my sleep form – it doesn't make any sense.

Last night: I went to bed at one o'clock, fell into a deep sleep, was woken by the boy after half an hour, had to lie down in his bed and didn't get to sleep before six o'clock. The night is so full of disturbances that my own treatment fades into the background. It's like trying to cure your own eating disorder during a famine. How could I even tell if the treatment was working?

The therapist looks at me. My turn. I look down at the form.

10th Nov.: Went to bed at 1 a.m. Woke up at 1.30 a.m. Woken up once for four-and-a-half hours. Got up at 7 a.m. Sleep efficiency: around 27?

'I've tried to fill in the form,' I begin. 'But the numbers are just a mess. When I go to bed at one o'clock, the kids wake up, so I don't get to sleep undisturbed. This treatment, which I've waited so long for, which I have such faith in, and which I'm so motivated to pursue – I'm going to have to drop it. It isn't about the pain, which is almost unbearable some days. It isn't even about what I'm putting my own family through. The treatment won't have any effect, it's as simple as that. Not with my home situation the way it is now.'

The regular pause follows before one of the therapists starts to speak.

'Sometimes that's how it goes. It just doesn't suit people. We have small children ourselves, so you have our deepest sympathies.'

On the way out one of the therapists grabs me.

'You can have another go,' he says, touching my shoulder lightly. 'Contact us when things have calmed down at home, okay?'

'Thanks,' I say, and go out into the November night.

Three whole weeks of wakefulness, sleep deprivation and struggles, all to no avail. But that night I sleep long and deep, and for the first time in many weeks, the children don't make a sound.

Treatment suspended.

Not cured.

I sleep and that's the only thing I care about right now.

DECEMBER

See you tomorrow

I

Doing the same thing every day is good for your sleep. Christmas celebrations are a disruption. In many ways, it's a choice between letting yourself be disrupted or not; between hurling yourself into life or trying to maintain control. On my bad days, it feels as if sleeplessness has robbed me of my ability to live a full life. If only I could sleep normally, I'd be a better father, a better husband, a better writer. I'd be happier and more active. But on the days when I'm in a state to lift my gaze, I see all the things I have: a family and friends; I've produced books and albums; I have a job. I've let myself be disrupted. I live a full life despite my sleeplessness. Maybe even *because of* my sleeplessness. Maybe it comes with the territory? The good days are so few, so dearly bought, that I value every single hour.

One evening just before Christmas, I crawl over the fence and take a bus into the city centre. Big Anders is in town and doesn't have much time, which suits me fine. One beer and then we can go our separate ways without the risk of having a night's sleep disrupted by too much alcohol. I tell him about my abandoned treatment. We meet rarely as we live on different sides of the country and both have kids and jobs. But Big Anders is familiar with my sleep problems. He asks me when I started sleeping badly. When I came to Oslo, I replied. When I stopped studying and started working.

'No,' he says. 'That's not right.'

'What do you mean?'

'You used to complain about not sleeping long before that.'

'Did I?'

'You were already sleeping badly in Bergen.'

I don't dig any deeper, thinking that he can't possibly know more about my insomnia than I do. We change the subject, drink our beers and then it's time for him to head off. On my way home I think about what he said. When did I actually start to sleep badly? I'd forgotten the trip to New York and how badly I slept then. And there was that summer of heartbreak. But these were isolated incidents, I think, as I crawl back over the fence. The insomnia came later. Didn't it?

Can I trust the story I am telling?

It is now more than sixteen years since I first went to the doctor with my sleep difficulties. I got sleeping pills. The pills stopped working and I set out on the long round of alternative treatment methods. The years passed. It got worse. I went to the doctor again, got pills again, and when the pills didn't work I started on the same round of alternative treatment methods again.

It's incredible that I don't remember all the things I've tried, and it's incredible that I find hope in the same hopeless efforts once again. I'm a man walking in circles around the wilderness, but because I can't see any other solutions, because I have no destination, I prefer to continue wandering around and around. I *want* to walk around in circles. After all, it feels better than stopping dead.

All the insomniacs I've spoken to seem to be trudging around in the same circle. Njål, Ingrid, Markus, Stian and the other sleepless people I've been in contact with. They seek out the same remedies over and over again, and they never make any noticeable difference – and this despite the fact that science and the sleep scientists of the world, *agree on what the best treatment is*. It's a hard task and it works for many people but not for all – it's no miracle cure – but it is something people can continue working with, maybe for the rest of their lives. Cognitive behavioural therapy. This is what science has identified as the answer. And it has been the obvious answer since the early 2000s – ironically enough, precisely the period in which I have suffered from this problem. And even more ironically, this answer turned out to have its headquarters right across the street from my home.

Why didn't I know this – after turning my life upside down in search of sleep? After trying to learn everything there is to be learned about sleep and sleep problems and how to treat insomnia?

But even more importantly: why didn't all the doctors I've visited over sixteen years know about this treatment? Why is it always pills or nothing? Indeed, why, whenever I've told a doctor about my sleeplessness, has it always seemed as if I was the first person to come to them with this ailment? If several hundred thousand Norwegians are suffering from insomnia, it is remarkable that the system society has built to handle and treat people with health problems is surprised by it.

'Despite international consensus that non-medical interventions, preferably CBTi, should be the first choice for the treatment of insomnia,' runs the *National Recommendation for the Study and Treatment of Insomnia* from 2018, 'major challenges remain when it comes to making this available on a sufficiently large scale.'

Sleep scientist Håvard Kallestad is more forthright when I speak to him about this treatment. 'We have a very widespread public health problem that seems only to be increasing among Norwegians, and a clear recommendation for a treatment that *almost nobody receives*,' he says. 'Within the field it is absolutely clear that the treatment is the best treatment we currently have. But few health personnel receive training or have sufficient knowledge about this.'

II

Sleep is still a mystery to most people. We spend one-third of our lives in this state, but have no idea what happens when we sleep, nor what causes the failure when sleep is denied us. My friends – most of them parents who are responsible for their children's health – sometimes talk on the subjects of disease and contagion with the air of experienced brain surgeons, sharing the knowledge they have acquired from doctors' appointments, Wikipedia and elsewhere. But when it comes to sleep, we're fumbling in the dark. We have *no idea* what brings sleep, we do not understand why it fails to come, but we become increasingly desperate. So, we approach sleep and sleep deprivation like a religion. Knowledge gives way to faith and desperation. Sleep is not a mystery and nor is sleeplessness. Insomnia is a public health problem suffered by every tenth adult in the Western world. Diminished quality of life, sick days, increased health risk – a vicious circle that can lead to depression and other disorders. Young people fail to get qualifications because of sleep problems. Today we are many. Tomorrow we shall be more.

I have another chat with Stian, the sleepless social worker student.

'Do you think your depression was the result of your sleep difficulties or vice versa?' I ask.

'They're interlinked,' Stian says. 'The fact that I can't sleep is part of a larger, complex mental health problem. But I have a New Year's resolution: I'm going to start going to bed and getting up earlier. I'm going to put away my laptop and mobile phone in the evenings and start reading again. Spending time on the internet is a way of switching off and stopping my thoughts buzzing. But at the same time, I know it isn't great for my sleep.'

I don't ask whether he's checked out the treatment I told him about last time we spoke because then he'll ask how *my* treatment went, and I don't have a good answer.

One evening, I get in touch with Markus again; it's ten o'clock and he's home from work. I wonder how he's been getting on with sleep since we last spoke, and he says it's going better. But the help has come at other people's expense. His father has had problems with sleep lately, so his GP prescribed him melatonin. And there was a trickle-down effect.

'Dad got melatonin on prescription, and I tried a bit of that. It's worked surprisingly well. I go to sleep more quickly and wake up without any side effects in the morning. So I think I'll ask the doctor for the same stuff. It's totally harmless because after all melatonin is something the body produces itself. If I take a pill a day that helps me to… well, at any rate, it works.'

III

New Year's Eve. Our family gets dressed up, packs sparklers in a rucksack and then drives across town to the friends we're celebrating the early part of the evening with. It's a cold, clear night, and the city is black and white beneath the darkness and the snow. The mild weather of the previous days has left a layer of shining ice upon the ground and when the first rockets explode against the sky I see their colours and light reflected in its sheen. After eating dinner and lighting the sparklers, the kids start to get tired and at around ten o'clock we leave the party. Far too early for us adults, of course, but well past bedtime for our two-year-old boy, who falls asleep in the car.

Our five-year-old now brushes her teeth and goes to the toilet on her own, and next autumn she'll be starting school. After she's got herself ready for the night, we go into her bedroom together. She undresses, then I pull her nightie over her head and bundle her up in her duvet. I read a bit from a book and we talk about the day that's just ended. There's no question of turning off the light: she has to have at least three lamps on if she's going to fall asleep. I let her have her way; I'll have to teach her about light and circadian rhythm when she gets a bit older. Or maybe not. For now, she seems to sleep well at night. Sleep is a gift, and so long as she has this gift, I don't want to do anything to disrupt it.

This particular night is special: the last of the old year and the first of the new. Maybe we'll wake her at midnight to watch the fireworks or maybe she'll be woken by the noise.

'Now you need to sleep,' I say. 'Now it's time to shut your eyes. Good night.'

Then I sit at the end of her bed. This is our arrangement at the moment. Before, I used to go into our bedroom, which is right beside hers and let her fall asleep by herself. For a short period, we could even sit upstairs in the living room while she lay down here alone. Then we had to come down and sit in the chair at her bedside. Now we're back at the foot of the bed. Tonight, I won't negotiate; I just want her to fall asleep as quickly as possible. She doesn't understand this herself, but if she can only get enough sleep, her tomorrow will be saved.

But tonight it doesn't work. She's restless, tossing and turning in her bed. I hear her whisper to herself, scratch herself, change position. Outside there are bangs, sometimes nearby, sometimes far away.

'Dad,' she says. 'I can't sleep.'

She should have fallen asleep long ago, so I do what I know works best: I lie down beside her and let her rest on my shoulder. She's still fidgety.

'Have you got any tricks for falling asleep?' she asks.

'Find a comfy position,' I say. 'Try and think of something nice you've done. Then breathe in and out slowly, listening to your own breath.'

At last, she seems to find peace. I feel her head grow heavier upon my shoulder and soon she stops fidgeting. Then I get up slowly. She turns over onto her side.

'See you tomorrow,' she murmurs after me.

'See you tomorrow.'

I go up to the first floor. I don't know what the night holds, but I try not to think about it too much.

Line falls asleep before midnight. I crack open a soft drink and watch the fireworks for a couple of minutes. Read New Year texts from friends and family, which become fewer and fewer as the years go by, and answer a few of them. Shall I stay up? Shall I go to bed?

A new year, my seventeenth as an insomniac. I will try the Sleep School treatment one more time; I feel certain that it will work: I just have to wait until my children sleep more continuously at night – then I can fix my own sleep.

I go to bed at one o'clock and can't sleep. Go back up and lie on the sofa, watch a bit of TV, but sleep evades me. Outside, it has fallen quiet. I look at the clock. 2.30 a.m.

See you tomorrow, we say to each other. What we really mean is: see you after sleep. When we are robbed of sleep, we lose both our tomorrow and our yesterday – the now simply goes on and on, and we go around in circles. Humans are fragile creatures. We are trapped in our own experience and are not designed to absorb everything around us. If we do, we go under. Because sleep isn't just rest, it is also a hiatus. It is the full stop at the end of a long sentence, the yearned-for cut in the film. It is mercy: one thing can end and something new can begin.

When I started writing this book I wanted to talk about my own sleepless life, but I discovered a bigger story, about a species that doesn't want to go to bed. Humans have made the waking portion of their existence less and less optimal for sleep. TV, smartphones, tablets, alcohol, coffee, nightlife, late and heavy dinners, entertainment, after-parties – it's as if everything modern humans enjoy most in the whole world must come at the expense of sleep.

Over the past five hundred years, we have broken away from the natural development of sleep that has prevailed as long as our species has lived beneath the sun. What's more, we have made a virtue of forcing ourselves out of bed early in the morning. This virtue leaves no room for the fact that we, as individuals, have completely different needs when it comes to sleep. The two-year-old who needs twelve hours' sleep has to go to kindergarten so that his parents can work. The teenager who is genetically predisposed to become more tired later in the evening and struggles to get up early has to go to school from morning onwards. Adult humans who need anything from four to ten hours' sleep a night, some of them early birds, others night owls, all have to get up and go to work. And thus, we live out our days, some rested, others fit to drop.

If prolonged continuous sleep was what once made us human – where are we heading now?

I know I'll get by; insomnia colours my life but has not conquered me. Yes, I'm afraid. But I have never stopped hoping. It's like being in a carriage on a train that has stopped in the middle of a desolate stretch, but you remain seated. You are restless and impatient, but you never leave the train; you stay in your seat because you know that sooner or later the train will slowly start to move again and your journey will resume.

AFTERWORD

How to live better with serious sleep disorders

I think offering superficial advice on how to combat insomnia doesn't just mislead insomniacs – it also disconnects them from an understanding of their own problems. Insomnia is inextricably linked to the individual's own lifestyle and psyche. Quite simply, to *who you are*.

Moreover, insomnia is a serious, complicated and long-lasting condition. Many of the sleepless people I have met have suffered from sleep problems their entire life. If that's the case, a list of quick fixes isn't going to be much help. So I had actually decided not to include such a list. Indeed, this book was a reaction against all the sleep advice.

But I've learned along the way that it is useful to meet other sleepless people and exchange experiences. The burden becomes lighter to carry. You understand your own problems a bit better. And even if you don't eliminate your sleep problems, it may still be useful to learn what helps and what doesn't. I live better with my sleep problems today than I did in the early years. So, if it's possible to boil down all that I have experienced and learned over many years as a sleepless person, why not try to share it – in as simplified and comprehensible a way as possible? Here are my ten pieces of advice:

1. The most important issue is not how long but *how* you sleep. Just a few hours of deep continuous sleep are better than a long night with many interruptions.

2. Don't lie to yourself. If you want better sleep, you need to know what your sleeping pattern is first. So: write down how you sleep. How long? How many times do you wake up?

3. Do what you like. Don't try to adapt your sleep to other people. Don't worry too much about keeping everybody happy. It doesn't work.

4. Log off. Sit down or go out and build a snow castle. The art of falling asleep is intimately connected to the art of being present. At least that's what I think.

5. Fixed routines are good. Find some that suit you. Don't make too much of a big deal out of it.

6. You are responsible for your own life. Continue to make decisions, big and small.

7. Do try and find out what you are *actually* afraid of when you're afraid of not sleeping. It may help to talk to somebody who knows you well. Like, what are you up to? Think it and it grows. Say it out loud and it diminishes.

8. Desperation is the lifeblood of all mental disorders. All these rules, routines and thoughts about getting sleep can contribute to heightened self-consciousness and, as a result, pressure. So: don't try too hard.

9. Cognitive behavioural therapy is the only treatment that I can say with certainty has helped me. The most important things I learnt were: get up at the same time every morning. Don't lie in bed longer than you usually

sleep. For example: you sleep five hours every night and want to get up at seven every morning. You are not allowed to go to bed until 1.30 a.m. in the morning and must get up at seven o'clock – no matter what. If you don't sleep in that time period, you must get up and try again later. Stay awake until the next night. It's tough to start off with. But it works for most people.

10. Live your life. I know that isn't easy.

ACKNOWLEDGEMENTS

This book couldn't have happened without the help and support of others.

I would like to thank all the people with sleep problems whom I've been in contact with for giving me full access to their own problems.

I wish to thank all the sleep experts who have devoted time to my project, especially sleep scientists Børge Sivertsen, Håvard Kallestad, Nikolaj Kahn and Bjørn Bjorvatn, as well as specialist psychologist Lina Elise Hantveit and director research Ingeborg Hartz.

My thanks to Fritt Ord for supporting this project.

Thanks to my editor Mattis Øybo, for his patience, enthusiasm and alertness, and to all the other lovely, talented people at Tiden forlag.

Thanks to Morten Eikrem for reading, and for his medical expertise.

Thanks to Thomas Mala for reading and contributing along the way.

Thanks also to Liv Guneriussen, Caroline Nesbø Baker and Nils-Øivind Haagensen for their contributions and commitment.

I would also like to take this opportunity to thank everybody who tries every day with the best intentions to help everybody else to sleep better – whatever the method.

Finally, thank you to my nearest and dearest for holding out: Line, Johanne and Jørgen. Without you, I have nothing to stay awake for.

SOURCES

Ascher, R., *The Nightmare*, horror documentary (2015).

BBC The Inquiry *'Have We Always Felt This Tired?'* interview with Roger Ekirch (2018).

Berna, F., P. Goldberg, L. Kolska Horwitz, J. Brink, S. Holt, M. Bamford, M. Chazan, 'Microstratigraphic evidence of in situ fire in the Acheulean strata of Wonderwerk Cave, Northern Cape province, South Africa', article published by PNAS.org (15th May 2012).

Bjorvatn, B., *Bedre søvn* (Fagbokforlaget, 2nd edition 2015).

Bjorvatn, B., B. Sivertsen, S. Waage, F. Holsten, S. Pallesen, 'Nasjonal anbefaling for utredning og behandling av insomni' *SØVN* (2018).

Cioran, Emil, *A Short History of Decay* (1949).

Fisher, Teresa, 'Descartes' Sleeping Habits and the Theory of the Sleeping Mind' *medium.com* (2015).

Foster, R., *Why Do We Sleep?* Ted Talks lecture (2013).

Fougea, F., J. Guiot, *Premier Homme*, documentary (2017).

Furu, K., V. Hjellvik, I. Hartz, Ø. Karlstad, S. Skurtveit, H. Salvesen Blix, H. Strøm, R. Selmer, *'Legemiddelbruk hos barn og unge i Norge 2008–2017'* report published by the Norwegian Public Health Institute (2018).

Huffington, A., *The Sleep Revolution* (W. H. Allen 2016).

Knoph Vigsnæs, M., 'De søvnløse', article in *VG Nett* (2017).

Lahti ,Tuuli A., 'Transitions into and out of daylight-saving time compromise sleep and the rest-activity cycles' *BMC Physiology* (2008).

Moran, Lee, 'Chinese Football fan, 26, Dies after Going 11 Nights without Sleep…', *Daily Mail* (22nd June 2012).

Parkin, S., 'Finally, a Cure for Insomnia?', article published in the *Guardian* (15th October 2018).

Pallesen, S., B. Sivertsen, Inger H. Nordhus, B. Bjovatn, 'A 10-year trend of insomnia prevalence in the adult Norwegian population' article in *Sleep Medicine* (2013).

Poe, Edgar Allen, *The Premature Burial*, short story (1844).

Randall, David K., *Dreamland* (W. W. Norton 2012).

Regier, Willis G., 'The Philosophy of Insomnia' *chronicle.com* (2011).

Rowan, Karen, 'Lack of sleep may harm men's sperm', *livescience* (2013).

Sacks, Oliver, *Hallucinations* (2012).

Schmidt, R., 'Caffeine and the Coming of Enlightenment', *Raritan: A Quarterly Review* (2003).

Sivertsen, B., P. Salo, A. Mykletun, M. Hysing, S. Pallesen, S. Krokstad, Inger H. Nordhus, S. Øverland, 'The Bidirectal Association Between Depression and Insomnia: The HUNT Study' article published in *The American Psychosomatic Society* (2012).

Skard Heier, M., Anne M. Wolland, *Søvn og søvnforstyrrelser* (Cappelen Akademisk Forlag 2005).

Celmer, Lynn, 'Sleep deprivation disrupts regulation of body heat', article published on *sleepeducation.org* (2012).

Spilde Ingrid, 'Reinsdyr uten døgnrytme' *forskning.com* (2005).

Stevenson, S., *Sleep Smarter: 21 Essential Strategies to Sleep Your Way To a Better Body, Better Health, and Bigger Success* (Hay House UK 2016).

Tse, Vivian, 'Good Night's Sleep Key to Beauty', *thelocal.se* (2013).

van Sant, G., *My Own Private Idaho* (1991).

Walker, M., *Why We Sleep* (Penguin 2018).

Interviews:

Børge Sivertsen, sleep scientist.

Bjørn Bjorvatn, sleep scientist.

Håvar Kallestad, sleep scientist.

Ingeborg Hartz, director of research at Innlandet Hospital Trust.

Lina Elise Hantveit, specialist psychologist.

Various anonymous insomniacs.

ENDNOTES

1. Matthew Walker, *Why We Sleep* (Penguin, 2018), p. 283.

2. Walker, *Why We Sleep*, p. 286.

3. Ståle Pallesen, Børge Sivertsen, Inger Hilde Nordhus and Bjørn Bjorvatn, 'Ten-year trend of insomnia prevalence in the adult Norwegian population' *Sleep Medicine* (2013).

4. Bjørn Bjorvatn, *Bedre søvn* (Fagbokforlaget, 2nd edition 2015), p. 31.

5. Walker, *Why We Sleep*, p. 57.

6. Fred Fougea and Jeromé Guiot, *Premier Homme* (2017), French documentary.

7. Mona Skard Heier and Anne M. Wolland, *Søvn og søvnforstyrrelse* (Cappelen Akademisk Forlag 2005), p. 34.

8. In Roman mythology the god of sleep is Somnus.

9. David K. Randall, *Dreamland* (2012), p. 230.

10. Randall, *Dreamland*, p. 229.

11. Walker, *Why We Sleep*, p. 193.

12. Walker, *Why We Sleep*, p. 204.

13. Walker, *Why We Sleep*, p. 213.

14. Walker, *Why We Sleep*, p. 215.

15. Walker, *Why We Sleep*, p. 28.

16. Norwegian caffeine information, kaffe.no

17. Shawn, Stevenson, *Sleep Smarter: 21 Essential Strategies to Sleep Your Way to a Better Body, Better Health and Bigger Success* (Hay House UK, 2016), p. 7.

18. Stevenson, *Sleep Smarter*, p. 186.

19. Skard Heier and Wolland, *Søvn og søvnforstyrrelse*, p. 36.

20. Walker, *Why We Sleep*, p. 30.

21. Skard Heier and Wolland, *Søvn og søvnforstyrrelse*, p. 36.

22. Ingrid Spilde, 'Reinsdyr uten døgnrytme' (2005), forskning.no

23. Walker, *Why We Sleep*, p. 24.

24. Teresa Fisher, 'Descartes' Sleeping Habits and the Theory of the Sleeping Mind' *medium.com* (2015).

25. Emil Cioran, *A Short History of Decay* (1949).

26. Russell Foster, 'Why do we Sleep?' (2013) lecture on Ted Talks, https://www.ted.com/talks/russell_foster_why_do_we_sleep

27. Lee Moran, 'Chinese Football fan, 26, Dies after Going 11 Nights without Sleep…', *Daily Mail*, 22nd June 2012, https:www.dailymail.co.uk/news/

article-2660134/Chinese-football-fan-39-dies-
suffering-stroke-brought-staying-three-nights-
watch-live-World-Cup-coverage.html

28. Walker, *Why We Sleep*, p. 254.

29. Walker, *Why We Sleep*, p. 258.

30. Lynn Celmer, 'Sleep deprivation disrupts
    regulation of body heat', article published on
    sleepeducation.org (2012)

31. Walker, *Why We Sleep*, p. 174.

32. Walker, *Why We Sleep*, p. 178.

33. Karen Rowan, 'Lack of sleep may harm men's
    sperm', (2013), livescience. no website.

34. Vivian Tse, 'Good Night's Sleep Key to Beauty',
    (2013), *thelocal.se*

35. Walker, *Why We Sleep*, p. 140.

36. Walker, *Why We Sleep*, p. 147.

37. Walker, *Why We Sleep*, p. 148.

38. Walker, *Why We Sleep*, p. 150.

39. Børge Sivertsen, Paula Salo, Arnstein Mykletun,
    Mari Hysing, Ståle Pallesen, Steinar Krokstad,
    Inger Hilde Nordhus and Simon Øverland, 'The
    Bidirectal Association Between Depression and
    Insomnia: The HUNT Study' (2012), *American
    Psychosomatic Society*.

40. Walker, *Why We Sleep*, p. 79.

41. Walker, *Why We Sleep*, p. 94.

42. Walker, *Why We Sleep*, p. 243.

43. Bjorvatn, Bedre søvn (2015), p. 31.

44. Ståle Pallesen, Børge Sivertsen, Inger Hilde Hordhus and Bjørn Bjovatn, 'Ten-year trend of insomnia prevalence in the adult Norwegian population' (2013), *Sleep Medicine*

45. Walker, *Why We Sleep*, p. 244.

46. Interview with Bjørn Bjorvatn (2018).

47. Walker, *Why We Sleep*, p. 245.

48. Walker, *Why We Sleep*, p. 246.

49. Roger Schmidt, 'Caffeine and the Coming of the Enlightenment', *Raritan: A Quarterly Review*, (Rutgers University 2003).

50. Oliver Sacks, *Hallucinations* (2012).

51. Maria Knoph, Vigsnæs, 'De Søvnløse', (2019), *VG Nett*, https://wwwvg.no/spesial/2017/de-sovnlose/

52. Skard Heier and Wolland, *Søvn og søvnforstyrrelse*, p. 186.

53. Skard Heier and Wolland, *Søvn og søvnforstyrrelse*, p. 206.

54. Skard Heier and Wolland, *Søvn og søvnforstyrrelse*, p. 214.

55. Randall, *Dreamland*, p. 153.

56. Tuuli A. Lahti, 'Transitions into and out of daylight-saving time compromise sleep and the rest-activity cycles' *BMC Physiology*, (2008), https://bmcphysiol.biomedcentral.com/articles/10.1186/1472-6793-8-3

57. Walker, *Why We Sleep*, p. 269.

58. Walker, *Why We Sleep*, p. 270.

59. Walker, *Why We Sleep*, p. 269.

60. BBC *The Inquiry*, 'Have We Always Felt This Tired?', interview with Roger Ekirch (2018).

61. Randall, *Dreamland*, p. 30.

62. Francesco Bernal, Paul Goldberg, Liora Kolska Horwitz, James Brink, Sharon Holt, Marion Bamford and Michael Chazan, 'Microstratigraphic evidence of in situ fire in the Acheulean strata of Wonderwerk Cave, Northern Cape Province, South Africa,' *PNAS.org*, (15th May 2012).

63. Randall, *Dreamland*, p. 34.

64. Randall, *Dreamland*, p. 35.

65. Sivertsen B et al., 'Cognitive behavioral therapy vs zopiclone for treatment of chronic primary insomnia in older adult: a randomized controlled trial.' (2006) *JAMA*, 295 (24) pp. 2851–8.

www.sandstonepress.com

facebook.com/SandstonePress/

@SandstonePress